# Managing Hazards in the Transfusion Service

**Harold B. Anstall, MD**
Professor of Pathology, University of Utah School of Medicine
Medical Director, Transfusion Services, Associated Regional and University Pathologists, Salt Lake City, Utah

**Robert C. Blaylock, MD**
Assistant Clinical Professor of Pathology, University of Utah School of Medicine
Associate Director of Transfusion Services, Associated Regional and University Pathologists, Salt Lake City, Utah

**Catherine M. Craven, MD**
Associate Director of Laboratories, Primary Children's Medical Center
Salt Lake City, Utah

ASCP PRESS

American Society of Clinical Pathologists
Chicago

Acquisition and Development: Joshua Weikersheimer
Editor: Karen D. Johnson
Production Manager: Andrea Blumenfeld
Designer: Ophelia M. Chambliss-Jones
Cover Design: Andrea Blumenfeld
Marketing Representative: Shannon Hansford



Library of Congress Cataloging in Publication Data

Anstall, Harold B., 1932–
Managing hazards in the transfusion service/ by Harold B. Anstall, Robert C. Blaylock, Catherine M. Craven.
p. cm.
Includes bibliographical references and index.
ISBN 0-89189-324-5
1. Blood—Transfusion—Complications and sequelae. I. Blaylock, Robert C. II. Craven, Catherine M. III. Title.
[DNLM: 1. Blood Transfusion—adverse effects. WB 356 A624h]
RM171.A649 1992
615'.39—dc20
DNLM/DLC
for Library of Congress
91-44122
CIP



Printed in the United States of America.
97 96 95 94 93 5 4 3 2 1

# Contents

# ACKNOWLEDGMENTS

We wish sincerely to acknowledge the tireless and painstaking efforts of Ms. Kim Cash for her initial preparation of the manuscript, and Ms. Joan E. Robinson, Staff Associate, for her excellent achievement in the editing and final arrangement of the text for publication. We thank them not only for the excellence of their accomplishments but also for the tact and patience with which they handled the foibles of the various authors. We would also like to express our gratitude to Mr. Don Morse for his excellent preparation of the illustrations.

# Introduction

Blood transfusion has been a hazardous practice from its inception. Apart from the early and medieval attempts at infusion of blood (usually that of animals) into humans as a revitalizing procedure, which usually resulted in severe reaction or death, transfusion in a more modern sense began in the early 19th century. The British obstetrician Blundell, for example, attempted direct donor-to-recipient (arm-to-arm) transfusions of patients who were in severe shock following postpartum hemorrhage. He found from these experiments, however, that an appreciable proportion of them became desperately ill, often dying of what we now recognize to have been a hemolytic transfusion reaction.[1,2] Other clinicians of the 19th century, sporadically attempting direct transfusions of this sort for a variety of causes, encountered these same problems. It was apparent that the technique was very much a hit-and-miss affair with the potential of grave risk and even fatal consequences for the recipient, with no way to predict the outcome in advance.

In 1900, Landsteiner[3] discovered the ABO blood group system, which provided the solution to the puzzle surrounding the origin of the hemolytic transfusion reactions, thereby laying the foundation for compatibility testing, which followed in simple form a few years later.[4] During the last 4 decades, rapid advances in immunology and immunohematology of have greatly increased our understanding of the factors responsible for immediate and delayed hemolytic reactions. Also, the high levels of sophistication in antibody detection and antibody identification have greatly reduced the risk of such complications. Today, the small number of those reactions that continue to be seen are generally the result of human error. Even in such cases, improved methods of management have resulted in substantial reduction of dangerous complications. Other immunologically determined reactions involving white blood cells and platelets (eg, febrile responses and noncardiogenic pulmonary edema) are recognized and can be prevented in large measure by appropriate technology, which excludes unnecessary leukocyte-related antigen from many products being transfused. Moreover, a better understanding of the mechanisms of such reactions enables adequate clinical management to be applied in most cases. Of greater practical importance nowadays is the association of transmissible infectious agents with transfusion practice. For example, the relationship between the administration of blood-derived products and subsequent occurrence of jaundice was first recognized in 1883, when an outbreak of what we call today "hepatitis" followed a smallpox vaccination using lymph derived from humans.[5] In the early decades of the 20th century, outbreaks of jaundice occurred frequently in conjunction with the treatment of syphilis by organic arsenicals. It was not long before a link was established between the repeated use of inadequately sterilized needles and the appearance of jaundice. Such cases were ascribed to the transmission of an infectious agent. The disease was identified as either "homologous serum jaundice" or "serum hepatitis" even though little or nothing was known of the nature of the agent responsible.[6]

Hepatitis, first recognized around 1943 as a complication of transfusion of blood products, sometimes developed several months after exposure. The coidentity of "homologous serum jaundice" and transfusion-related hepatitis was thus established, and the condition was ascribed to an uncharacterized viral agent.[7] To make a long story short, it is now well known that at least 2 basically unrelated viral agents—hepatitis B and hepatitis C—account for the overwhelming majority of such cases that result from transfusion of blood products. Modern methods of immunologic testing for hepatitis B and C markers have provided valuable screening methods for the elimination of potentially infectious donors, thus greatly improving the safety of the blood supply now available. These relationships and the potential linkage between transfusion and the transmission of other viral agents, such as cytomegalovirus (CMV), are discussed in detail in this text.

The most dramatic developments of recent years in the field of transfusion-transmissible disease (TTD) have occurred in tandem with the discovery of human retroviruses as the causal agents of the acquired immunodeficiency syndrome (AIDS) and human T-cell leukemia. The now-exploding worldwide AIDS epidemic, while threatening whole populations, has brought about an acute consciousness of the transmissibility of this condition through certain blood products and underscores the necessity of meticulously screening donors who provide such products. The advent of accurate and sensitive immunologic tests to detect human immunodeficiency virus (HIV) and, more recently, human T-cell lymphotropic virus-I (HTLV-I), has greatly narrowed the risk from transmission of these agents to recipients of blood products. Understandably, owing to the severe and often fatal consequences of such transmission, the public has become extremely sensitive to the potential risk. This ever-increasing sensitivity has elicited an appropriate response: the meticulous screening of blood donors historically, physically, and immunologically for the potential presence of the viral agents responsible and for behavorial attributes that are associated with a high risk of infection by these agents.[8]

Because of the great and expanding concern, among medical and paramedical professionals as well as the public at large, it is necessary in a monograph of this sort to emphasize the potential infectious complications of blood transfusion. By the same token, it is also necessary to indicate the positive aspects of this important branch of medicine; namely, although conservatism in practice is amply justified, the safety of transfusion practice is steadily increasing. This is due to our cognizance of potential risks and to the development of sensitive screening and confirmatory procedures for most of the infectious agents capable of causing problems. In the overall perspective, transfusion of blood products should be viewed in much the same way as major surgical procedures: it should not be undertaken lightly and without sound clinical justification. Furthermore, it should be withheld where such indications are not present.

This monograph is designed to give the clinician, the transfusion service physician, the nurse, and the medical technologist a reasonably comprehensive survey of the potential hazards of transfusion and to arrange these in a sequence that, at the very least, is logical. This survey attempts to follow the full course of transfusion practice, beginning with risks to the blood donor, which range from potential sources of error in the processing, laboratory handling, labeling, and distribution of blood products, to those hazards directly involving a recipient. These in turn are considered under appropriate etiologic categories: immunologic, infectious, and mechanical. It is hoped that this approach will create the impression of a "flow of hazards," which will further define the scope and limits of things that may go wrong involving the donor, the laboratory handling of blood products, and the recipient. The emphasis will be substantially on the issue of prevention and protection of both donors and patients. Although the text contains some necessary theoretic material, we have attempted to limit its inclusion to the extent that it is sufficient for the intelligent understanding of the subjects under discussion. Our emphasis, therefore, favors the practical approach to a full comprehension of the material presented.

Whereas some of the material described in this work can be pooled together from other published sources, we hope that by arranging the material in this particular sequence, real benefits will accrue to those involved in practical blood transfusion work whether performing as clinician, blood bank worker, technologist, or nurse. Conscious of the fact that such works are often significantly dated by the time they are published, we have attempted to emphasize certain general principles of transfusion practice that are concerned more with the maintenance of high standards of safety, rather than the minute and mutable details. It is hoped that this objective will be achieved.

Harold B. Anstall
Professor of Pathology and Medical Director, Transfusion Services
University of Utah Medical Center
Salt Lake City, Utah

## References

1. Harvey W. De Motu Cordis, 1628. Cited by: Petz LD, Swisher SN, eds. Blood Transfusion in Clinical Practice. New York, NY: Churchill-Livingstone; 1981.
2. Fletcher JL, Zmiewski CM. Introduction in Immunohematology. New York, NY: Appleton-Century-Crofts; 1972.
3. Landsteiner K. Uber Agglutinationscheinungen normalen Menschlichen Blutes. Wien Klin Wochenschr. 1901;14:1132.
4. Anstall HB. Transfusion in historical perspective. In: Anstall HB, Urie PM. A Manual of Hemotherapy. New York, NY: Churchill-Livingstone; 1986:1.
5. Lurman A. Eine Ikteroepidemie. Klin Wochenschr. 1885;20:20.
6. Zuckerman AJ. TV chronicle of viral hepatitis. Hygiene. 1979;54:111. Abstract.
7. Beeson PB. Jaundice occurring one to four months after transfusion of blood or plasma. JAMA. 1943;121:1332.
8. College of American Pathologists Conference XVI. AIDS and the pathologist. General review; 1990.

## CHAPTER 1

# DONOR-RELATED HAZARDS

## REACTIONS DURING BLOOD DONATION

The acquired immunodeficiency syndrome (AIDS) has dramatically changed the practice of transfusion medicine during the past decade.[1,2] The recognition of the transfusion of blood products as a major risk factor for the transmission of the human immunodeficiency virus (HIV) made the safety of the blood supply a concern of medical personnel and the general public. A tremendous amount of research and effort have been devoted to reducing the risk of HIV and hepatitis transmission through blood. Changes have been implemented in donor screening procedures and laboratory testing of blood, which are designed to identify persons at risk for transfusion-transmitted disease (TTD) and to prevent potentially contaminated units from entering the blood supply. Despite the impact TTDs have had on the collection and processing of blood, other areas of danger or liability encountered in transfusion medicine cannot be overlooked. Policies and procedures regarding blood collection must not only be designed to provide the safest blood product for the recipient but also should maximize donor safety as well.

### Pathophysiology of Donor Reactions

Reaction rates during blood donation have been reported to occur with an incidence of approximately 5% but vary considerably.[3-8] Donor reactions have been associated with physiologic factors, psychologic factors, and a combination of both. A blood donation consists of approximately 450 mL, which represents about 10% of the average donor's blood volume. This amount can increase to 13% of total blood volume in donors who weigh the minimum required, 50 kg (110 lbs). Although there is evidence for the correlation of blood volume donated and donor reaction rate, by far the majority of donors are able to compensate for this blood loss by increasing venous tone and reducing the amount of blood in the venous system. Blood becomes available for the maintenance of normal cardiac output and blood pressure. Circulatory compensatory mechanisms are such that significant changes in blood pressure and heart rate are not usually encountered with the donation of a unit of blood.[8] If tachycardia is detected with orthostatic hypotension, the reaction may be due to reduction in blood volume. Bradycardia is normally associated with vasovagal reactions. It is important to try to differentiate between vasovagal reactions and reactions due purely to hypovolemia, but both can be contributing factors depending on the individual. The 2 reaction types are treated differently, and it might become necessary to treat hypovolemia with intravascular crystalloid solution if the reaction is prolonged or progresses in intensity.

A "vasovagal attack" is mediated through the autonomic nervous system with far-reaching effects. These reactions appear to begin in the hypothalamus, are transmitted through the autonomic nervous system, and result in inappropriate reductions in heart rate and blood pressure. Additional symptoms include sweating, nausea, vomiting, incontinence, unconsciousness, and, in severe instances, seizures. Donors can also hyperventilate in response to the discomfort and anxiety provoked by the reaction. Hyperventilation can result in increased removal of $CO_2$ from blood with an ensuing respiratory alkalosis. This alkalosis causes plasma proteins to have an increased affinity for free serum calcium. This reduction in free serum calcium can result in involuntary muscle contraction and increase the severity of a reaction.

## Factors Associated With Donor Reactions

Many risk factors have been associated with increased chance of encountering a donor reaction. Some of these risk factors are characteristic of the donor (physiologic and psychologic), while others relate to the physical environment in which the donor is placed both before and during the phlebotomy procedure. Characteristics involving the donor include previous donor reactions, first donation, donor personality, nervousness, young age, high heart rate, and low body weight. The influence of initial blood pressure on reaction rates has varied.[3,4,8-12] Generally, investigators have found higher reaction rates among women.[3] Some factors believed significant by experienced phlebotomists, but not confirmed as independent risk factors in studies, include hunger and fatigue.[8] The first of these can be avoided by feeding the donor prior to phlebotomy. The practice of feeding donors, however, may be unwise if done directly prior to phlebotomy. The nourishment will not provide any immediate benefit, while increasing the risk of aspiration if the individual experiences a donor reaction and vomits. The fatigue factor is not as easily avoided, and it is the opinion of many that donors should not be deferred on the basis of fatigue alone.[8]

Phlebotomists should project confidence in their abilities and have interpersonal skills that enable them to put donors at ease and reduce apprehension. An experienced phlebotomist with an outgoing, cheerful personality can be instrumental in reducing reaction rates.[12] This factor is important since it can be influenced to some degree by personnel training. Other environmental factors include long waiting lines, extremes in temperature, and a noisy, crowded collection site. Donors who witness others experiencing a donor reaction are at increased risk for having a reaction themselves. It is therefore prudent to isolate donors recovering from a reaction.

## Types of Donor Reactions

Donor reactions have been broken into 3 main categories for ease of recognition and implementation of treatment. A mild reaction consists of signs and symptoms including complaints of anxiety and feelings of warmth, pallor, perspiration, dizziness, lightheadedness, hyperventilation, and nausea with or without vomiting. Treatment of a mild reaction includes cessation of the phlebotomy procedure, placing a cold pack on the forehead or back of the neck of the donor, placing the donor in the Trendelenburg position, and loosening any tight clothing. Vital signs should be measured at regular intervals. Hyperventilatory alkalosis should be avoided by having the donor breathe into a paper bag, hold his/her breath, or take long, deep, slow breaths. If the donor does not respond quickly, additional medical help should be summoned. Donors should never be left unattended.

A moderate reaction includes all the signs and symptoms as described for a mild reaction with progression to periods of unconsciousness, hypotension, shallow respirations, and reduction in heart rate. Treatment of a moderate reaction include those already listed for a mild reaction with continued measurement of all vital signs except temperature.

The last category of donor reactions are severe reactions, which are rare. A reaction is classified as severe when a donor is observed to have a convulsion or seizure. Convulsions can occur when the vasovagal reaction reduces cerebral blood flow to the point where ischemia develops. Spasms can be precipitated from the respiratory alkalosis caused by hyperventilation. Maintenance of an airway may be necessary. Help should be called for immediately. In the event a donor undergoes an arrest, phlebotomists must be able to perform cardiopulmonary resuscitation. At no time should a phlebotomist leave the donor. Other individuals in the donor area should be instructed to obtain medical assistance as necessary.

All donor reactions should be reported to the medical director of the transfusion service. Any donor undergoing more than a mild reaction should have a complete history of the reaction recorded including degree of severity, duration, and a record of any necessary treatment. A donor who has experienced a reaction, and recovered while in the presence of donor center personnel, is still at risk for problems after leaving the donation site. The donor should be moved by wheelchair if further examination or treatment is deemed necessary or escorted to his/her car with arrangements made for someone to chauffeur the donor home. These actions are intended to prevent any further injury from trauma during a second episode of syncope.

## Iron Deficiency in Blood Donors

### A Brief Review of Iron Balance

A long-standing area of concern for blood collection agencies is the effect of frequent whole blood donation on the iron balance in an individual. Iron deficiency anemia can result from repeated donation of whole blood. Unfortunately, the entire blood supply of this country is provided by a small minority of the population. This places blood banks in the position of asking for multiple donations from a relatively small number of individuals. Guidelines are in place that are designed to prevent the inappropriate collection of blood from iron-depleted donors, but these guidelines are not 100% sensitive in screening out individuals at risk for iron deficiency anemia.

Iron is necessary for the normal production of heme-containing compounds, which are chiefly hemoglobin and myoglobin. The total iron content of men is approximately 50 mg/kg, whereas that of women is 35 mg/kg.[13] This difference is believed to be because of the high prevalence of iron deficiency in women (in developed countries up to 20% of adult women and 50% of pregnant women).[13] Red blood cells at the end of a 120-day life span are removed from the circulation by the reticuloendothelial system. Iron is extracted from hemoglobin and carried in plasma by the transport protein transferrin to the bone marrow. In the marrow, the iron is incorporated into hemoglobin prior to the release of young red blood cells (RBCs) into the peripheral circulation. Iron is efficiently recycled. Iron losses occur only when cells are lost from the body during the normal turnover of various epithelial layers, during pregnancy, or from RBC loss of any kind (eg, menstruation, blood donation). Men and nonmenstruating women require approximately 1 mg/day of iron to maintain balance. This requirement is doubled for menstruating women and can be 3 to 4 times higher during pregnancy. Iron levels are controlled by regulating the amount of iron absorbed from the diet. Absorption rates increase or decrease depending on the level of iron stores.

### Effect of Blood Donation on Iron Stores

The donation of a unit of blood results in a loss of between 200 and 250 mg of iron. This may not represent a significant loss to a man with 1 g of storage iron, but it is significant compared to the 200 to 400 mg of iron stores found in many menstruating women. Repeated blood donation is associated with decreased marrow hemosiderin and plasma ferritin levels.[14,15,18,21,22] Hemoglobin or hematocrit values are the only laboratory parameters determined before donation. While this information prevents the removal of blood from anemic individuals, hemoglobin or hematocrit levels do not correlate with iron stores and may be normal when iron stores are depleted.[14-18] A serum ferritin level is the best test for predicting iron stores,[19,20] but a rapid test methodology that would make donor screening practical is not available. It is not surprising that reduced iron stores are found more often in menstruating women who donate blood compared to men or postmenopausal women.[14] The total number of units donated in a lifetime is not a good predictor of iron depletion, but the frequency of donation (number of units per year) does correlate with iron stores. Men are able to donate up to 5 or 6 units a year with relatively little problem, but iron depletion is common in menstruating women donating more than 1 to 2 units a year. Variables that enable individuals to donate blood frequently include large body size and a superior diet (increased kilocalories, iron, and ascorbic acid ingestion).[23]

### Prevention of Iron Deficiency

Oral iron supplementation has been demonstrated as an effective method to prevent iron depletion in blood donors, and even casual ingestion of iron can reduce the incidence of iron deficiency greatly.[14,24-27] The routine administration of iron to individuals who are not anemic can be controversial because of the potential for masking pathologic blood loss (eg, gastrointestinal malignancy) or accentuating iron overload in individuals with undiagnosed hemochromatosis. A donor group in whom iron supplementation may be considered is women of childbearing age. This group has high iron demands secondary to losses incurred during pregnancy and menstruation. A once-daily dosage of a supplement that contains 40 mg of elemental iron will allow premenopausal women to donate as frequently as men (up to 5 units/year).[25,26] Menstruating women not taking oral iron supplements should probably be advised not to donate blood more than 1 to 2 times a year. All patients giving autologous blood should take iron up to the anticipated time of surgery and beyond, depending on net blood loss and discharge hemoglobin values. A blanket policy increasing the interval between whole blood donation (currently 56 days) could reduce the risk of iatrogenic iron deficiency but may also severely reduce the available blood supply by unnecessarily limiting donation from men and nonmenstruating women.

### Screening for Anemia

Obtaining hemoglobin levels prior to blood donation does not prevent the collection of blood from individuals with marginal iron stores, but it will prevent the inappropriate bleeding of anemic donors. Many donor centers use a copper sulfate screening test, which is a qualitative method for determining a minimum hemoglobin level. A drop of blood must sink through a solution of copper sulfate, with a known specific gravity, within 15 seconds. Hemoglobin concentrations are higher when collected from earlobe puncture compared to fingerstick samples. The specific gravity of the copper sulfate solution must be adjusted upward if earlobe samples are used for screening.[28] Donors who fail the copper sulfate screen should have a microhematocrit performed since the gravimetric test can underestimate hemoglobin values.[29] Some blood centers prefer to perform microhematocrit determinations on all donors since the copper sulfate test can overestimate hemoglobin levels as well.[14] Donors deferred because of anemia need to be advised to obtain proper medical follow-up. Unless it is clear the cause of the anemia is due to repeated blood donation (eg, frequent donations from a menstrual woman), a pathologic cause for the anemia must be considered with appropriate work-up directed by the donor's personal physician.

## Autologous Donation

The practice of individuals predepositing blood intended for transfusion into themselves prior to procedures in which blood loss is anticipated is not a new concept in transfusion medicine. Autologous blood transfusion was initiated as a means of preventing transfusion-associated hepatitis and became widely used after the recognized transmission of HIV through blood products. This discovery made physicians and the general public fearful of the blood supply. Many procedures involving the screening of potential donors and laboratory testing have been put into place to improve the safety of homologous blood. Regardless of the number of implemented safeguards, transfusion will always carry risks. Potential complications following transfusion of blood products include transfusion-transmissible diseases, transfusion reactions, alloimmunization (ie, HLA, platelet-specific or RBC antigens), and rarely, graft-vs-host disease (GVHD). Because of these risks, it is clear that in the majority of cases that autologous blood is the safest blood available to the patient. In general this is true, but autologous blood cannot be collected and transfused without consideration being given to the clinical condition of the patient and/or the method used to obtain the autologous product. There are 4 methods to obtain autologous blood: 1) predeposit; 2) preoperative collection with hemodilution; 3) intraoperative salvage; and 4) postoperative salvage.[30] All patients undergoing an elective surgical procedure where blood use is anticipated should be examined regarding which autologous blood strategy is best. Failure to inform patients of alternatives to homologous blood can result in litigation. Many patients can predeposit their entire blood requirements prior to surgery, but some patients may need an autologous strategy designed that includes a combination of these 4 collection methods. Autologous blood has proven efficacious and safe for a broad variety of patient demographics and clinical situations.[31-36]

**Predeposit**

The most common method for obtaining autologous blood is by predepositing blood prior to the anticipated date of use. Rigid criteria that apply to homologous donors are relaxed for autologous donors. Guidelines for the collection of autologous blood are set by individual institutions. American Association of Blood Banks (AABB) recommendations state that autologous blood should not be collected when the hematocrit is less than 33%.[33] The phlebotomy schedule is set by the blood bank physician in consultation with the patient's physician and should not occur more frequently than every 72 hours (preferably 1 week between donations) with the last donation not less than 72 hours before anticipated use.

No age restrictions are placed on autologous blood donors. A study evaluating the ability of children (8–18 years of age) to provide autologous blood demonstrated a donor reaction rate (all mild reactions) comparable to rates found in first-time adult donors.[37] The amount of blood collected was adjusted for body weight with the majority of patients donating 1 to 2 unit equivalents collected at weekly intervals, but as many as 5 unit equivalents were collected. An impressive 88% of the children in the study supplied their entire blood needs and had no exposure to homologous blood.

Regular donors older than 65 years of age have been shown to be excellent sources of blood with donor reaction rates similar to a cohort of younger donors.[38] A study comparing reaction rates among autologous donors of all ages found the elderly autologous population to actually have the fewest complications.[39] Age alone should not be a deciding factor in determining the eligibility of a patient for autologous predeposit.

The use of autologous blood collection during pregnancy is a source of debate.[40,41] Studies have been published demonstrating that blood can be collected safely from pregnant women, but the absolute risks to mother and baby have not been ascertained.[42-45] The largest study evaluating pregnant autologous donors demonstrated no statistically significant difference in donor reaction rates compared to a homologous population, even though 66% of the pregnant women were first-time blood donors.[42] All of the reactions were classified as mild. No increased rates of infant morbidity or mortality have been reported, but the possible effects on a fetus of a moderate or severe donor reaction, with concomitant decreases in blood pressure and cardiac output, have not been determined.

Women have high iron demands during pregnancy. The average pregnancy results in a net decrease of 680 mg of maternal iron stores.[13] This requirement is not equally prorated over the entire pregnancy, with the largest demands being in the third trimester. The timing of much autologous donation also occurs during this portion of pregnancy, with each unit donated increasing iron loss by 200 mg. Collecting 3 units of blood will almost double the iron lost during the average pregnancy. The effects this increased loss has on mother and infant have not been adequately studied and must be considered when contemplating an autologous program for pregnant women, including the optimal time for blood collection.

Pregnant patients with the diagnosis of placenta previa appear to be a group who benefits from precollection of autologous blood. Reports have demonstrated that between 33% and 80% of patients with placenta previa receive autologous blood transfusions.[42,49,50]

The transfusion rates for pregnant patients have been reported to be less than 3%.[46-48] Based on this figure it is obvious that the routine collection of autologous blood from pregnant patients will result in the majority of the blood being wasted. A defined set of clinical circumstances, which select pregnant patients with increased risk for needing transfusion at delivery, should be established by the hospital's transfusion service in coordination with the obstetrics department. These criteria should reduce the amount of unindicated and wasteful blood donation by pregnant women.

The safety of autologous blood collection in other "high-risk" patients, such as those with coronary artery disease, valvular heart disease, and congenital heart disease, has been evaluated.[51] No severe untoward effects were encountered while these patients donated; however, people with unstable angina or left mainstem coronary artery disease were not included in the study. Patients with unstable angina and symptomatic valvular disease, especially aortic stenosis, are probably not good candidates for donation. Blood should not be obtained from patients with symptomatic disease without consultation with the patient's physician. Aggressive blood centers may collect blood from these patients under conditions of heavy monitoring and at a site capable of handling any adverse reactions to the donation. With recent improvements in the screening of homologous donors and expanded laboratory testing of products, one must weigh the risk to the patient from donating autologous blood against the risks of receiving a homologous product.

Laboratory testing of autologous blood remains an area of transfusion medicine that is devoid of uniform guidelines. The Food and Drug Administration (FDA) requires that autologous blood be tested for HIV-1 antibody and HBsAg and that serologic testing for syphilis be performed. No testing is necessary, however, if the autologous unit is to be used in the institution in which it is collected. Limited or no testing of autologous units can reduce processing costs, and the facility collecting the blood does not have to make decisions regarding the handling of units testing positive for infectious disease markers. Problems can arise if the site of a patient's surgery is unexpectedly changed. Units with no testing cannot be moved to the new surgical site, and partially tested units may or may not be accepted, depending on the policies of the blood bank where the procedure will take place. Many blood centers process autologous products in an identical fashion to homologous blood, since exceptions to normal processing protocol are impractical to implement. Decisions must now be made regarding which units with positive markers, if any, will be allowed in the blood bank for transfusion. Some blood banks will make any unit available for transfusion, arguing that although patients may be positive for HBsAg, they are not infected with HIV and should be able to receive their own blood. Other blood banks believe that the risk of transfusing an autologous product to the wrong patient does not justify the entrance of HIV-positive or other viral marker–positive units into the blood bank. The risk of exposing laboratory personnel to potentially infectious units is also considered. Generally, units with an increased alanine aminotransferase (ALT) or positive results for HBcAb are allowed into most blood banks for use as autologous products.

Unused autologous blood products may be placed into the general blood inventory if the donor meets all the criteria set forth for regular blood donors. The decision to "crossover" autologous products is left to individual blood banks. Debate exists regarding the safety of autologous products for use in the general blood inventory.[52] An argument against crossover of autologous products is that autologous donors are not true volunteers and have incentive to donate that involves avoiding homologous blood. A study evaluating the rate of transfusion-transmitted disease in recipients of crossover autologous blood has not been published. Many institutions have found the number of unused autologous units meeting regular donor criteria, and not at the end of the unit outdate, an insignificant addition to the general blood inventory. The increased record keeping and clerical logistics involved in crossover of autologous blood are difficult to justify for a small number of units.

### Intraoperative Salvage

The intraoperative collection and reinfusion of blood during surgical procedures has proven to be an effective method of reducing homologous blood requirements when used alone or in combination with predeposited autologous blood. This method can be used for many surgeries including orthopedic, vascular, and cardiac procedures.[52] The only absolute contraindication to the use of blood salvaging is contamination of the surgical site with malignant cells or bacteria. The washing process will not remove either of these contaminants. Collection of deleterious substances and their subsequent systemic dissemination must be avoided. Most intraoperative harvest equipment involves the collection, washing, and reinfusion of RBCs,[53-57] but some procedures involve filtration alone.[55,58]

The transfusion service should give advice regarding the procedures developed for the collection of salvaged blood, the personnel performing the collection, and which type of system is used.

**Postoperative Salvage: "Shed Blood"**

Autologous blood transfusion can involve blood that has been collected from surgical drains postoperatively. This autologous source of RBCs is often referred to as "shed blood." Mediastinal drainage following cardiothoracic procedures is a common source of shed blood,[59,60] but the collection of blood from joint spaces following orthopedic surgical procedures is becoming more popular. Current AABB standards mandate that blood collected postoperatively be infused within 6 hours of the time collection was initiated.[61] The standards also state that tissue debris and other sterile contaminants may necessitate special processing such as washing. Devices for the collection of "shed blood" are available, which allow the blood to be collected and infused through a 40-μm filter without the blood leaving the patient's room or being placed in a transfer pack. Proponents of this technique cite advantages of nursing convenience and the infusion of plasma proteins. Indeed, few patient complications have been described using this type of system, but shed blood that is not washed contains activated components and/or by-products of the complement, soluble coagulation, and fibrinolytic systems that have the potential of causing harm to the patient. The debate regarding the need to wash shed blood continues.[62,63]

Fibrin degradation products (FDPs) are potent inhibitors of fibrin formation and platelet function.[64-66] Unwashed salvaged blood contains high concentrations of by-products of the fibrinolytic system.[59,67,68] Infusing inhibitors of fibrin formation and platelet function in theory could result in delayed postsurgical hemostasis and an increased RBC loss. Benefits of the autologous product can be partially offset by infusing high concentrations of FDPs. The presence of FDPs in shed blood also indicates that the fibrinolytic system has been activated. Pouring the plasmin contained in drainage blood directly into a patient could also cause inappropriate fibrinolysis and fibrinogenolysis. The addition of unnecessary plasmin will magnify the anticoagulant effects of the FDPs and cause further delays in obtaining hemostasis. Salvaged blood is defibrinogenated.[68] Transfusing an unwashed product will not supply the patient with clotting factors or any substance that could be beneficial in maintaining balance between hemostasis and thrombosis. On the contrary, unwashed shed blood may contain activated products of the coagulation system that could be deleterious to the patient.

An in-house study at the University of Utah was conducted to evaluate the in vitro characteristics of washed vs unwashed shed blood from

7 patients undergoing total knee replacement. The unwashed supernatant demonstrated the ability to cause in vitro fibrin formation when used in place of tissue thromboplastin to initiate a prothrombin time. The washed supernatant did not initiate clotting. Obviously any substances that can initiate clotting in an in vitro system could also initiate clotting in vivo if introduced into the circulation in large-enough concentrations. Statistically significant reductions in prothrombin times have been reported in a group of patients receiving unwashed shed mediastinal blood when compared to a group receiving a washed product. Reduced prothrombin times are consistent with hypercoagulable states.

A delicate balance exists between hemostasis and thrombosis, which, if disrupted, can result in varying degrees of coagulopathy. In addition to possible perturbation of the coagulation system, concerns exist regarding the effects of leukoattractants and activated components of the complement system and the potential for lung damage caused by these contaminants.[68-70] Although few adverse effects have been described after the infusion of shed blood, the time, effort, and money involved in washing blood salvaged postoperatively seem worthwhile until the in vivo effects of shed blood have been clearly delineated.

### Preoperative Hemodilution

Autologous blood may be collected just prior to a surgical procedure by replacing the volume of blood collected with an equivalent amount of sterile intravenous solution. The amount of blood collected varies depending on the patient's hematocrit, size, and clinical condition, but it usually ranges between 1 to 2 units. The blood collected can remain in the operating room at 20° to 24°C for up to 6 hours and has some advantages over stored autologous blood in that platelet function and all clotting factors remain viable. It is believed that oxygen delivery to tissues is not compromised after RBC removal.[71] The reduced oxygen-carrying capacity of blood is compensated by the increase in cardiac output that occurs secondary to reductions in blood viscosity. After hemodilution, lower-hematocrit blood is lost during surgery and the previously collected high-hematocrit blood can be transfused when the procedure is near completion and hemostasis is achieved.

The blood bank must be involved in preparing protocols for the proper collection and labeling of blood collected in an operating room, even if the procedures are performed by an anesthesiologist or other surgical personnel.

## Directed Donation

The public fear of HIV transmission from an infected unit of blood has prompted many patients to select specific blood donors who are thought to be at no risk of being infected with HIV or some other transfusion-transmissible disease. No evidence exists supporting the theory that patients are better at selecting low-risk individuals than blood bank professionals,[72] and directed donation is a topic of much debate.[73,74] The use of directed donation is accepted for a limited number of clinical situations. These include collecting platelets from family members of patients who are refractory to platelet transfusion secondary to alloantibodies directed against HLA or platelet-specific antigens. Another situation involves the collection of rare blood types from family members of a patient needing compatible blood. Many pressures are placed on blood banks from patients and clinicians to provide directed donations for routine blood transfusion. The competitive climate in medicine has led many hospitals to provide directed donation for fear of losing patients to a hospital already providing the service. Most physicians would agree that directed donations should not be used as a marketing tool or instituted secondary to the fear of a lawsuit from a patient denied directed blood, but reality is such that these factors do enter into the decision to initiate or maintain directed donation programs.

**Pros & Cons**

The most persuasive argument against the use of directed donations involves the theory of directed donations being less safe than homologous blood because of the pressure or possible coercion placed on the donor to donate. Directed donors with risk factors for transmitting disease can be placed in an awkward situation since anonymity is lost, and questions will be asked by the patient if the blood is not available for transfusion (removing the effectiveness of confidential unit exclusion). While this is a concern, directed donations have not been shown to have a higher rate of viral marker positivity compared to first-time homologous donors.[72] Proponents of directed donation argue that by knowing the patient, a directed donor may be more thorough during the screening procedure for fear of harming the patient. Patients should provide a list of individuals from whom they would like donations. This will prevent the unsolicited donation from people not clearly requested from the patient.

The confidentiality of a directed donor can be a concern if the unit tests positive for a viral marker or if the recipient develops a transfusion-transmissible disease. A system should be established that reduces complications related to confidentiality, including the rapid notification of the donor concerning positive viral marker test results. When directed donors are asked to explain to family or friends why their donation was not available, they can state "the blood was not compatible for transfusion." When patients request directed donations they should sign a consent form explaining that while blood types between the donor and recipient may be the same, this does not guarantee compatibility between the donor's blood and the patient's blood. "Incompatible for transfusion" can include unexpected RBC antibodies found in the patient's serum or the finding of a positive viral marker. A patient should rarely need specifics regarding lack of compatibility. Directed donors need information explaining how their confidentiality is compromised when compared to a regular homologous donor, and this education process should be documented for the protection of the blood collection agency.

Other arguments against directed donation include the increased cost of paperwork and the logistics involved in tracking a unit and assuring its transfusion into the appropriate individual. Increased costs are also incurred if potential donors need to be typed prior to donation. A mathematical model evaluating the chances of finding a suitable number of directed donors for patients with different blood types and of varying ethnic backgrounds has been published.[75] First-degree relatives were demonstrated to be most likely to have compatible ABO groups. Blood collected for transfusion to first-degree relatives should be irradiated to eliminate the risk of graft-vs-host disease.

A woman should not receive blood from a man who could potentially father a child with the woman, or any of his family members, since presensitization to paternal RBC antigens carries a small risk of causing hemolytic disease of the newborn.[76] Likewise, blood should not be transfused from a bone marrow donor into a potential recipient of the marrow because engraftment could be jeopardized due to presensitization.

### Effect on Autologous Programs

A transfusion service with a directed donation program should not become lackadaisical regarding the promotion of autologous blood practices. Even after patients are told no scientific evidence exists demonstrating superior safety of directed donation over regular homologous blood, some patients still believe directed donations are as safe as autologous blood.[77] Evidence also exists that patients utilizing a mixture of autologous and directed donations to meet anticipated blood needs do not have reduced exposure to homologous blood when compared to patients meeting the requisite number of units entirely with autologous donation.[78] It appears physicians tend to order less homologous blood and tolerate lower hematocrits for patients who participate in an autologous program only.

## Special Donor Complications Relating to Apheresis

Apheresis involves separation and collection of a desired portion of whole blood while returning the remaining components to the patient or donor. Apheresis is effective in treating patients with various clinical diseases, such as the removal of plasma containing pathologic autoantibodies from a patient with myasthenia gravis. Apheresis is also used for the routine production of blood products, especially platelet concentrates. Early in the practice of transfusion medicine, plasmapheresis was accomplished by collecting a volume of blood, allowing the RBCs and plasma to separate by gravity, removing the plasma, and reinfusing the RBCs back to the patient. This process is accomplished now by the mechanical centrifugation of blood with separation into various components depending on specific gravity. This differential centrifugation will layer blood components in order of decreasing density: RBCs, granulocytes, monocytes, lymphocytes, platelets, plasma. These layers are not absolute, and some overlap exists.

Apheresis machines use either intermittent or continuous-flow technology. Intermittent machines require only one site of venous access. A specified volume of blood is collected into a container and centrifuged. The desired component is removed, and the remainder of the blood is reinfused through the catheter from which it was obtained. The process is repeated until the desired amount of plasma, or other blood component, has been collected. The extracorporeal volume of the system should not exceed 15% of the blood volume of the patient or donor. Different bowl sizes are available depending on the calculated blood volume. Continuous-flow systems are available that infuse and withdraw blood simultaneously, but access to 2 venous sites is necessary. Both methods have unique advantages and disadvantages.

Donors participating in plateletpheresis programs can experience donor reactions similar to those seen in whole blood donation, but additional problems can be encountered. Apheresis donors who donate more frequently than the 56-day interval necessary for whole blood donation are at theoretic risk for depletion of various blood components. An example of a clinical circumstance that requires a donor to participate in frequent collection is the need to provide HLA-matched platelets for a patient refractory to platelet transfusion secondary to HLA alloimmunization. The minimum interval between apheresis donations must be at least 48 hours. In addition to time limitations, additional laboratory monitoring of donors is necessary if collection is more frequent than that recommended for whole blood.

## Depletion of Blood Components

The amount of plasma collected from donors must be kept below 1000 mL per week.[79] Studies evaluating the removal and recovery rates of various plasma constituents during plasma exchange, using albumin as a replacement fluid, have demonstrated different patterns depending on the analyte measured. Progressive decreases in immunoglobulin levels, complement, and cholesterol can be seen.[80] Transient reductions in coagulation factors and antithrombotic substances such as protein C and antithrombin III occur, but complications secondary to thrombosis or hemorrhage are rare.[81,82] These decreases were demonstrated after therapeutic procedures and should not be encountered in apheresis donors in whom plasma collection is limited. Nevertheless, frequent apheresis donors should have total protein levels above 60 g/L (6 g/dL) and serum protein electrophoresis or quantitative immunoglobulins evaluated at least every 4 months.

Red blood cell losses in apheresis donors should be monitored, kept at a minimum, and should never exceed 200 mL in a 56-day period. Hemoglobin or hematocrit determinations should be made prior to each donation.

Current methodology does not permit the collection of granulocytes in quantities capable of depleting marrow reserves. However, the removal of lymphocytes after repeated thrombocytapheresis procedures can be significant.[83-86] A single thrombocytapheresis procedure can remove between 2 x $10^9$ and 4 x $10^9$ lymphocytes, which represents approximately one third of circulating lymphocytes.[79,87,88] The number of lymphocytes lost during apheresis is highly dependent on the type of machine used and can be greatly reduced (0.35 x $10^9$ per procedure) with some continuous-flow methods.[89] In addition to quantitative losses, decreases in various in vitro lymphocyte assays were also noted, including T-cell subpopulations, T4:T8 ratios, and lymphocyte response to various mitogens.[83] This study involved apheresis technology with large lymphocyte losses (2–4 x $10^9$ per procedure) in donors averaging 72 plateletpheresis procedures during an 8-year period.

A short-term study that removed a mean of 41 x $10^9$ lymphocytes from donors during a 12-day period demonstrated no decreases in absolute lymphocyte counts and no abnormal in vitro qualitative tests.[86] HLA-matched apheresis platelets are necessary for patients refractory to platelet transfusions secondary to HLA alloantibodies. An individual donor may be asked to provide many apheresis donations over a short period if limited donors are available with the HLA type of a patient needing matched-platelet transfusion. This study suggests that short-term removal of large numbers of lymphocytes may not be detrimental to the donor.

Deliberate lymphocyte depletion has been attempted experimentally for the treatment of autoimmune diseases, such as rheumatoid arthritis. Lymphocytopenia that results in immunosuppression can be achieved using apheresis or thoracic duct drainage. The exact lymphocyte loss needed to cause lymphocytopenia is not known but is generally thought to be between 5 and 40 x $10^{10}$ cells over a period of a few days.[84] One study subject developed an intestinal fistula 2 weeks after an appendectomy, and another developed herpes zoster of the seventh cranial nerve. These incidents occurred 9 and 6 months, respectively, after the study was performed. The relation of these incidents to the lymphapheresis procedures is not known. These losses are far more than would be expected from the routine production of apheresis platelets regardless of the instrumentation used for collection, especially if donation intervals are reasonable.

There have not been reports of an increased incidence of opportunistic infections in apheresis donors. An increased frequency of life-threatening opportunistic infections has been reported in patients with rapidly progressive glomerulonephritis undergoing therapeutic plasmapheresis to remove circulating immune complexes.[90] These patients not only had underlying renal disease but were also being treated with cytotoxic agents and steroids. The long-term risks of repeated lymphocyte harvest to healthy apheresis donors are not known. In theory, the possibility of iatrogenic immunosuppression from removal of lymphocytes, immunoglobulins, and complement exists. When possible, thrombocytapheresis procedures should be performed with instruments that limit lymphocyte depletion. If necessary, absolute lymphocyte counts (ALC) can be monitored and a donor deferred if the ALC drops below 1200/μL.[79,84]

Advancement to more aggressive chemotherapy regimens for the treatment of leukemia during the 1960s resulted in a group of patients who routinely became thrombocytopenic. Platelet transfusions proved efficacious in preventing spontaneous hemorrhage in this group of patients.[91] Platelets can be prepared from units of whole blood or by apheresis. Platelets prepared by apheresis have the advantage that a therapeutic dose can be obtained from a single donor. Multiple donors are required if a therapeutic dose of platelets is prepared from single collections of whole blood. The risk of a patient developing a transfusion-transmissible disease can be reduced by a factor of 6 to 8 by using platelets prepared by apheresis. The reduced risk of transmitting disease and the need to provide HLA-matched platelets has resulted in more thrombocytapheresis procedures.

The template bleeding time will increase when platelet counts drop to below 100 x $10^9$/L (100,000/$mm^3$), but significant bleeding following trauma does not generally occur until counts fall to below 50 x $10^9$/L (50,000/$mm^3$). Reducing the platelet count of a donor to a marginal level of safety is undesirable and, in practice, rarely encountered. A thrombocytapheresis procedure harvests 4 to 7 x $10^{11}$ platelets, which results in a 20% to 30% drop in the donor's pre-apheresis platelet count.[84,87,88] Criteria should be used that will minimize the chances of dropping the platelet count to below 100 x $10^9$/L (100,000/$mm^3$). Approximately 4 to 7 days are necessary for platelet counts to return to pre-apheresis levels.[92,94] If an individual is required to donate more often than once a week, a platelet count should be performed and found to be greater than 150 x $10^9$/L (150,000/$mm^3$) before the procedure is started.[84] Deferring donors with platelet counts below this level will result in only 1.3% of donors having a postapheresis platelet count below 100 x $10^9$/L (100,000/$mm^3$) and will not result in unreasonable deferral rates.[92] Donors participating in plateletpheresis at regular whole blood intervals do not need additional laboratory testing.

**Citrate Toxicity**

The production of blood components using apheresis requires the manipulation of whole blood in an extracorporeal system. The blood must be safely anticoagulated to avoid the formation of emboli, which could be deleterious to the donor or patient in the case of a therapeutic procedure. Solutions using various concentrations of citrate are the most widely used anticoagulant for apheresis. Citrate binds calcium, making it unavailable for normal platelet aggregation or the soluble coagulation system.[95]

Donor or patient symptoms related to hypocalcemia can result if citrate is infused too rapidly. These symptoms include circumoral tingling, nausea, vomiting, gastrointestinal cramping, substernal chest pain, carpopedal spasms, and rarely, overt tetany.[96] Hemodynamic changes can be seen with prolongation of the QT interval on electrocardiogram (ECG).[97,98] Symptoms can occur during apheresis procedures or during rapid and massive infusion of citrated blood products.[99]

The frequency and severity of symptoms are related to the citrate concentration of the anticoagulant solution, the delivery rate of citrated product, and the duration of the procedure.[96] Careful attention to these factors can reduce donor discomfort and potential danger.[100] Generally, donors complain of mild symptoms, such as perioral tingling, when ionized calcium levels drop 20% to 30% of pre-apheresis levels, but symptomatology increases greatly when levels drop 35% or more.[98,101] Ionized calcium levels will not always correlate with symptoms or electrocardiogram changes.[98] Citrate delivery rates ranging between 1.0 and 1.8 mg/kg per minute will result in a 20% to 35% reduction in ionized calcium. Citrate flow rates at this level usually limit donor symptomatology to parasthesias but are high enough to allow adequate blood flow rates for efficient collection of platelets. Donor discomfort can be controlled by reducing citrate flow rates or by supplementation with oral calcium. Rarely, severe citrate reactions will necessitate the discontinuance of the apheresis procedure with the administration of intravenous calcium gluconate.

Therapeutic plasma exchange theoretically should frequently cause symptomatic hypocalcemia, since significant quantities of calcium are removed with unwanted plasma, and citrate is present, reducing free calcium levels. However, calcium levels are well maintained during therapeutic plasmapheresis.[102] Studies evaluating calcium homeostasis during plasma exchange have demonstrated that patients with normal parathyroid function have a rapid compensatory increase in N-terminal parathormone, which helps to maintain calcium levels. Hypocalcemia is not encountered as often as one might predict, but several other factors can exacerbate citrate toxicity during therapeutic plasma exchange and must be considered if a patient is symptomatic.

Fresh frozen plasma (FFP) is used as a replacement fluid in the treatment of thrombotic thrombocytopenic purpura. The citrate contained in the FFP can be significant when added to the citrate used routinely in the procedure. This additive effect can increase the potential for citrate toxicity and complications related to hypocalcemia any time FFP or another blood product collected in citrate is administered concurrently or in conjunction with the apheresis procedure.

Citrate is normally metabolized rapidly in the liver. Patients with impaired hepatic function may not be able to metabolize citrate efficiently and are at increased risk for toxicity. Any underlying disease process causing inherently low calcium levels necessitates close monitoring of ionized calcium during therapeutic procedures. Patients or donors who become anxious and apprehensive during a procedure, and begin to hyperventilate, can have a physiologic decrease in free calcium. Hyperventilation results in lowered plasma P-$CO_2$ levels and increased blood pH. Plasma proteins more effectively bind calcium at alkaline pH. While total calcium remains the same, free calcium is greatly reduced and the actions of citrate will be augmented. Efforts to return the donor/patient to a slow, steady respiratory pattern should be initiated when signs of agitation and hyperventilation begin. Having the donor consciously change his/her breathing pattern can help increase P-$CO_2$ levels and reduce the likelihood of carpopedal spasm.

## Complications Associated With Leukapheresis

Granulocyte transfusions have been shown to be effective in granulocytopenic patients with acute infection.[103,104] Recommendations for the use of granulocytes in adults include use in a patient with a good chance of bone marrow recovery, an absolute neutrophil count at least below $0.5 \times 10^9$/L (500/$mm^3$), and strong evidence of infection not responding to antibiotics.[105,106] The prophylactic use of granulocytes has not been shown to be effective.[107] Other problems associated with granulocyte use include difficulty in harvesting large numbers of neutrophils and the logistic problems resulting from the short shelf life of the product. Despite the proven efficacy of granulocyte transfusions, improvements in chemotherapeutic protocols and antibiotic use have almost eliminated the use of granulocyte transfusions in adults.

Granulocyte transfusions still play a role in the treatment of neonatal sepsis.[108,109] Neonatal sepsis occurs in up to 1 to 3 per 1000 live births[110] and can be associated with high degrees of morbidity and mortality. The reasons for the poor outcome in septic neonates include the following: 1) the low number of stem cells per kilogram of body weight, which results in low granulocyte production; 2) the inability to increase granulocyte production when challenged with a bacterial infection; 3) the poor response of neonatal granulocytes to chemotactic stimuli; 4) reduced phagocytosis capabilities; and 5) depression in oxygen-dependent, bacterial-killing mechanisms.[111] Providing adult granulocytes without qualitative defects can significantly increase survival in cases of neonatal sepsis. It is also possible to harvest granulocytes from adults in high enough numbers to be effective in neonates. Exact dosages have not been defined, but a study transfusing $10^9$ neutrophils (irradiated to prevent GVHD) per kilogram of body weight every 12 hours until neutropenia was no longer present was effective.[108] Many neonates will require only 1 transfusion.

Granulocyte products are made using apheresis technology. Harvesting adequate numbers of granulocytes can be difficult and is complicated because RBCs and granulocytes are in adjacent layers during differential centrifugation and some overlapping of the 2 cell populations exists. Methods used to improve the quantity and selectivity of granulocyte harvests include stimulating donor neutrophilia with the administration of steroids or by enhancing the separation of RBCs and granulocytes with the use of a RBC sedimenting agent.

Steroids are effective in raising peripheral granulocyte counts in donors if given several hours prior to donation. Any donor with health conditions that can be aggravated by steroids should not be used as a neutrophil donor. These conditions include peptic ulcers, glaucoma, and diabetes.[79] Short-term side effects of steroids, such as headache, palpitations, euphoria, and flushing, can also cause problems in donors.[79] The several-hour donor preparatory time may be available for the rarely encountered adult treatment protocol but is not realistic when providing granulocytes to a septic infant. Such a medical emergency requires the preparation and transfusion of the product in the shortest possible time, and donor preparatory time simply is not available.

Hydroxyethyl starch (HES) was originally developed as a plasma expander but also causes RBC rouleaux formation and is useful in increasing granulocyte yields during apheresis procedures.[102] Although the use of HES greatly improves the efficiency of granulocyte collection, HES is associated with some side effects. Hydroxyethyl starch has been implicated as causing allergic reactions including donor complaints of itching and sneezing with some reactions becoming anaphylactoid in nature.[112] Of more importance are the predicted side effects of HES relating to its original use as a plasma expander. A study evaluating the cumulative effects of HES in donors after 4 consecutive days of infusion demonstrated significant levels of HES 7 days after the last dose was given.[113] The average increase in plasma volume was approximately 1 L and correlated with an increase in HES levels. Twenty-four hours after the last dose was given, the majority of donors still had at least a 500-mL expanded plasma volume. Concurrent with increases in plasma volume were decreases in hematocrit, hemoglobin, total protein, and albumin. Donors complained of headache and swollen hands, but no cases involving shortness of breath or orthopnea were noted. The short-term, repetitive use of a granulocyte donor should be discouraged. If this type of donation is believed to be necessary, or serial therapeutic leukapheresis procedures are contemplated, the potential complications secondary to progressive plasma expansion must be considered. Since HES remains in plasma for a considerable period of time, plasma expansion can be minimized if HES is used on an intermittent basis or in progressively smaller daily doses. Hydroxyethyl starch has been associated with a case of lichen planus,[114] but the cause and effect was not proved, and lichen planus has been described in donors not receiving HES.[115]

Filtration leukoapheresis is a methodology once used for the production of granulocyte products but has been replaced with differential centrifugation procedures. Some unusual donor reactions have been reported with its use, including priapism in men, pelvic pain in women (described as being similar to uterine contractions), tenesmus, urgency, and some nausea.[116] A couple of theories were proposed for the reported cases of priapism. The first involves the activation of complement by the filtration process. These activated components of the complement system (ie, C5a) in turn cause leukostasis in the veins draining the corpus cavernosum. An alternate theory involves venous occlusion from platelet aggregates induced during heparin-mediated thrombocytopenia. Heparin was used as an anticoagulant in filtration procedures.

### Allergic Reactions Related to Ethylene Oxide Sterilization

Allergic reactions to ethylene oxide gas have been reported during apheresis.[117,118] Ethylene oxide is used to sterilize not only apheresis software harnesses but many medical instruments made of plastic that can be destroyed by the high temperature and humidity encountered in an autoclave. Periorbital edema, conjunctival itching, chemosis, coryza, tearing, facial flushing, abdominal cramping, diarrhea, urticaria, epigastric pain, and chest heaviness are all symptoms described with ethylene oxide allergic reactions.[117] Although severe morbidity and mortality have not been encountered secondary to ethylene oxide sensitivity during apheresis, serious

## References

1. Zuck TF. Legal liability for transfusion injury in the acquired immunodeficiency syndrome era. Arch Pathol Lab Med. 1990;114:309.
2. Willett DE. The duty to warn about transfusion risks. Arch Pathol Lab Med. 1989;113:307.

3. Callahan RC, Edelman EB, Smith MS, et al. Study of the incidence and characteristics of blood donor "reactors." Transfusion. 1963;3:76.
4. Poles FC, Boycott M. Syncope in blood donors. Lancet. 1942;2:531.
5. Moloney WC, Lonnergan LR, McClintock JK. Syncope in blood donors. N Engl J Med. 1946;234:114.
6. Ruetz PP, Johnson SA, Callahan R, et al. Fainting: a review of its mechanisms and a study in blood donors. Medicine. 1976;36:363.
7. Subcommittee of the Blood Transfusion Research Committee. Fainting in blood donors. Br Med J. 1944;1:279.
8. Tomasulo PA, Anderson AJ, Paluso MB, et al. A study of criteria for blood donor deferral. Transfusion. 1980;20:511.
9. Greenbury CL. An analysis of the incidence of "fainting" in 5,897 unselected blood donors. Br Med J. 1942;1:253.
10. Graham DT Prediction of fainting in blood donors. Circulation. 1961;23:901.
11. Brown H, McCormak P. Analysis of vasomotor phenomena (faints) occurring in blood donors. Br Med J. 1942;1:1.
12. Ogata H, Iinuma N, Nagashima K, et al. Vasovagal reactions in blood donors. Transfusion. 1980;20:679.
13. Wintrobe MM, ed. Clinical Hematology. 8th ed. Philadelphia, Pa: Lea & Febiger; 1981:153-163, 627.
14. Simon TL, Garry PJ, Hooper EM. Iron stores in blood donors. JAMA. 1981;245:2038.
15. Finch CA, Cook JD, Labbe RF, et al. Effect of blood donation on iron stores as evaluated by serum ferritin. Blood. 1977;50:441.
16. Gordeuk VR, Brittenham GM, Hughes MA, et al. Carbonyl iron for short-term supplementation in female blood donors. Transfusion. 1987;27:80.
17. Gordeuk VR, Brittenham GM, Bravo J, et al. Prevention of iron deficiency with carbonyl iron in female blood donors. Transfusion. 1990;30:239.
18. Pedersen NS, Morling N. Iron stores in blood donors evaluated by serum ferritin. Scand J Haematol. 1978;20:70.
19. Cook JD, Lipschitz DA, Miles LEM, et al. Serum ferritin as a measure of iron stores in normal subjects. Am J Clin Nutr. 1974;27:681.
20. Addison GM, Beamish MR, Hales CN, et al. An immunoradiometric assay for ferritin in the serum of normal subjects and patients with iron deficiency and iron overload. J Clin Pathol. 1972;25:326.
21. Fielding J, Karabus C, Brunstrom GM. Storage iron depletion in male blood donors: its significance for iron status in women. J Clin Pathol. 1968;21:402.
22. Hagberg B, Wallenius G, Wranne L. Latent iron deficiency after repeated removal of blood in blood donors. Scand J Clin Lab Invest. 1958;10:63.
23. Monsen ER, Critchlow CW, Finch CA, et al. Iron balance in superdonors. Transfusion. 1983;23:221.
24. Biregard G, Hogman C, Killander A, et al. Serum ferritin levels in male blood donors: relation to number of phlebotomies and iron supplementation. Vox Sang. 1978;34:65.
25. Simon TL, Hunt WC, Garry PJ. Iron supplementation for menstruating female blood donors. Transfusion. 1984;24:469.
26. Gordeuk VR, Brittenham GM, Bravo J, et al. Prevention of iron deficiency with carbonyl iron in female blood donors. Transfusion. 1990;30:239.
27. Gordeuk VR, Brittenham GM, Hughes MA, et al. Carbonyl iron for short-term supplementation in female blood donors. Transfusion. 1987;27:80.
28. Avoy DR, Canuel ML, Otton BM, et al. Hemoglobin screening in prospective blood donors: a comparison of methods. Transfusion. 1977;17:261.
29. Lloyd H, Collins A, Walker W, et al. Volunteer blood donors who fail the copper sulfate screening: what does failure mean, and what should be done? Transfusion. 1988;28:467.

30. The National Blood Resource Education Program Expert Panel. The use of autologous blood. JAMA. 1990;263:414.

31. Cowell HR, Swickard JW. Autotransfusion in children's orthopedics. J Bone Joint Surg. 1974;56:908.

32. Council on Scientific Affairs. Autologous blood transfusion. JAMA. 1986;256:2378.

33. Anderson BV, Tomasulo PA. Current autologous transfusion practices: implications for the future. Transfusion. 1988;28:394.

34. McVay PA, Hoag RW, Hoag MS, et al. Safety and use of autologous blood donation during the third trimester of pregnancy. Am J Obstet Gynecol. 1989;160:1479.

35. Mann M, Sacks HJ, Goldfinger D. Safety of autologous blood donation prior to elective surgery for a variety of potentially "high-risk" patients. Transfusion. 1983;23:229.

36. DePalma L, Luban NL. Autologous blood transfusion in pediatrics. Pediatrics. 1990;85:125.

37. Silvergleid AJ. Safety and effectiveness of predeposit autologous transfusions in preteen and adolescent children. JAMA. 1987;257:3403.

38. Pindyck J, Avorn J, Kuriyan M, et al. Blood donation by the elderly: clinical and policy considerations. JAMA. 1987;257:1186.

39. McVay PA, Andrews A, Kaplan EB, et al. Donation reactions among autologous donors. Transfusion. 1990;30:249.

40. Kruskall MS. The safety and utility of autologous donations by pregnant patients: pro. Transfusion. 1990;30:168.

41. Sayers MH. Autologous blood donation in pregnancy: con. Transfusion. 1990;30:172.

42. McVay PA, Hoag RW, Hoag MS, et al. Safety and use of autologous blood donation during the third trimester of pregnancy. Am J Obstet Gynecol. 1989;160:1479.

43. Kruskall MS, Leonard S, Klapholz H. Autologous blood donation during pregnancy: analysis of safety and blood use. Obstet Gynecol. 1987;70:938.

44. Milles G, Browne WH, Barrick RG. Autologous transfusions for elective cesarean section. Am J Obstet Gynecol. 1969;103:1155.

45. Herbert WNP, Owen HG, Collins ML. Autologous blood storage in obstetrics. Obstet Gynecol. 1988;72:166.

46. Palmer RH, Kane JG, Churchill WH, et al. Cost and quality in the use of blood bank services for normal deliveries, cesarean sections, and hysterectomies. JAMA. 1986;256:219.

47. Gibbs CE, Misenhimer HR. The use of blood transfusion in obstetrics. Am J Obstet Gynecol. 1965;93:26.

48. Kamani AA, McMorland GH, Wadsworth LD. Utilization of red blood cell tranfusion in an obstetric setting. Am J Obstet Gynecol. 1988;159:1177.

49. Malynn ER, Druskall MS, Nessen SL, et al. Analysis of autologous donations in pregnant women with placenta previa. Transfusion. 1988;6(suppl):34S.

50. Herbert WNP, Owen HG, Collins ML. Autologous blood storage in obstetrics. Obstet Gynecol. 1988;72:166.

51. Mann M, Sacks HJ, Goldfinger D. Safety of autologous blood donation prior to elective surgery for a variety of potentially "high risk" patients. Transfusion. 1983;23:229.

52. Silvergleid AJ. Preoperative autologous donation: what have we learned? Transfusion. 1991;31:99.

53. Mann DC, Wilham MR, Brower EM, et al. Decreasing homologous blood transfusion in spinal surgery by use of the cell saver and predeposited blood. Spine. 1989;4:1296.

54. Hall RI, Schweiger IM, Finlayson DC. The benefit of the Hemonetics cell saver apparatus during cardiac surgery. Can J Anaesth. 1990;37:618.

55. Hallett JW. Minimizing the use of homologous blood products during repair of abdominal aortic aneurysms. Surg Clin North Am. 1989;69:817.
56. Reddy DJ, Ryan CJ, Sheppard AD, et al. Intraoperative autotransfusion in vascular surgery. Arch Surg. 1990;125:1012.
57. Goulet JA, Bray TJ, Timmerman LA, et al. Intraoperative autologous transfusion in orthopaedic patients. J Bone Joint Surg. 1989;71-A:3.
58. Nakamura Y, Munetaka M, Toshima Y, et al. Comparative study of cell saver and ultrafiltration nontransfusion in cardiac surgery. Ann Thorac Surg. 1990;49:973.
59. Hartz RS, Smith JA, Green D. Autotransfusion after cardiac operation: assessment of hemostatic factors. J Thorac Cardiovasc Surg. 1988;96:178.
60. Schaff HV, Hauer JH, Bell WR, et al. Autotransfusion of shed mediastinal blood after cardiac surgery: a prospective study. J Thorac Cardiovasc Surg. 1978;75:632.
61. Widmann FK, ed. Standards for Blood Banks and Transfusion Services. 14th ed. Arlington, Va: American Association of Blood Banks; 1989:47.
62. Griffith LD, Billman GF, Daily PO, et al. Apparent coagulopathy caused by infusion of shed mediastinal blood and its prevention by washing of the infusate. Ann Thorac Surg. 1989;47:400-406.
63. Bergtson JP, Backman L, Stenquist O, et al. Complement activation and reinfusion of wound drainage blood. Anesthesiology. 1990;73:376.
64. Barnhart MI, Cress RL, Riddle SM. Influence of fibrinogen split products on platelets. Thromb Diath Haemorrh. 1967;17:78.
65. Kopec M, Budzynski SS, Wegrzyrowicz Z, et al. Studies on the mechanism of interference by fibrinogen degradation products with platelet function: role of fibrinogen in the platelet atmosphere. Thromb Diath Haemorrh. 1966;15:476.
66. Larrieu MJ, Rigollot C, Marder VJ. Comparative effects of fibrinogen degradation fragments D and E on coagulation. Br J Haematol. 1972;22:719.
67. Lawrence-Brown MMD, Couch C, Halliday M, et al. D-Dimer levels in blood salvage for autotransfusion. Aust N Z J Surg. 1989;59:67.
68. Hauer JM, Thurer RL. Controversies in autotransfusion. Vox Sang. 1984;46:8.
69. Bull MH, Bull BS, Van Arsdell GS, et al. Clinical implications of procoagulant and leukoattractant formation during intraoperative blood salvage. Arch Surg. 1988;123:1073.
70. Hangen DH, Stevens JH, Satoh PS, et al. Complement levels in septic primates treated with anti-C5a antibodies. J Surg Res. 1989;46:195.
71. Paty PSK, Shah DM, Chang BB, et al. Immediate preoperative phlebotomy with autologous blood donation for aortic replacement. Surg Gynecol Obstet. 1990;171:326.
72. Cordell RR, Yalon VA, Cigahn-Haskell C, et al. Experience with 11,916 designated donors. Transfusion. 1986;26:484.
73. Goldfinger D. Directed blood donations: pro. Transfusion. 1989;29:70.
74. Page PL. Directed blood donations: con. Transfusion. 1989;29:65.
75. Kanter M, Selvin S, Myhre BA. The probability of finding suitable directed donors. Arch Pathol Lab Med. 1989;113:174.
76. Kanter MH, Hodge SE. Risk of hemolytic disease of the newborn as a result of directed donations from relatives. Transfusion. 1989;29:620.
77. Chambers LA, Kruskall MS, Drago SS, et al. Directed-donor programs may adversely affect autologous donor participation. Transfusion. 1990;30:246.
78. Goodnough LT. Directed blood procurement does not benefit patients who are enrolled in an autologous blood predeposit program. Am J Clin Pathol. 1989;92:484.
79. Huestis DW. Risks and safety practices in hemapheresis procedures. Arch Pathol Lab Med. 1989;113:273.
80. Orlin JB, Berkman EM. Partial plasma exchange using albumin replacement: removal and recovery of normal plasma constituents. Blood. 1980;56:1055.

81. Sultan Y, Bussel A, Maisonneuve P, et al. Potential danger of thrombosis after plasma exchange in the treatment of patients with immune disease. Transfusion. 1979;19:588.
82. Mannucci PM, D'Angelo A, Vigano S, et al. Decrease and rapid recovery of protein C after plasma exchange. Transfusion. 1986;26:156.
83. Matsui Y, Martin-Alosco S, Doenges E, et al. Effects of frequent and sustained plateletapheresis on peripheral blood mononuclear cell populations and lymphocyte functions of normal volunteer donors. Transfusion. 1986;26:446.
84. Strauss RG, Huestis DW, Wright DG, et al. Cellular depletion by apheresis. J Clin Apheresis. 1983;1:158.
85. Senhauser DA, Westphal RG, Bohman JE, et al. Immune system changes in cytapheresis donors. Transfusion. 1982;22:302.
86. Blanchette VS, Dunne J, Steele D, et al. Immune function in blood donors following short-term lymphocytapheresis. Vox Sang. 1985;49:101.
87. Segel GB, Lichtman MA, Gordon BR, et al. Plateletpheresis residues: a source of large quantities of human blood lymphocytes. Transfusion. 1976;16:455.
88. Nusbacher J, Scher ML, MacPherson JL. Plateletpheresis using the Haemonetics Model 30 cell separator. Vox Sang. 1977;33:9.
89. Kurtz SR, McMican A, Carciero R, et al. Plateletpheresis experience with the Haemonetics Blood Processor 30, the IBM Blood Processor 2997, and the Fenwal CS-3000 Blood Processor. Vox Sang. 1981;41:287.
90. Wing EJ, Bruns FJ, Fraley DS, et al. Infectious complications with plasmapheresis in rapidly progressive glomerulonephritis. JAMA. 1980;244:2423.
91. Han T, Stutzman L, Cohen E, et al. Effect of platelet transfusion on hemorrhage in patients with acute leukemia. Cancer. 1966;19:1937.
92. Lasky LC, Lin A, Kahn RA, et al. Donor platelet response and product quality assurance in plateletpheresis. Transfusion. 1981;21:247.
93. Katz AJ, Genco, PV, Blumberg N, et al. Platelet collection and transfusion using the Fenwal CS 3000 cell separator. Transfusion. 1981;21:560 .
94. Huestis DW, Bove JR, Case J. Practical Blood Transfusion. 4th ed. Boston, Ma: Little, Brown & Co Inc; 1988:372-380.
95. Hastings B, McLean FC, Eichelberger L, et al. The ionization of calcium, magnesium and itrontium citrate. J Biol Chem. 1934;107:351.
96. Hester JP, McCullough J, Mishler JM, et al. Dosage regimens for citrate anticoagulants. J Clin Apheresis. 1983;1:149.
97. Bunker JP, Bendixen HH, Murphy AJ. Hemodynamic effects of experimental hypercitremia. Anesthesiology. 1967;28:510.
98. Landenson JH, Miller WV, Sherman LA. Relationship of physical symptoms, ECG, free calcium, and other blood chemistries in reinfusion with citrated blood. Transfusion. 1978;18:670.
99. Nealon TF, Ching NPH, Gibbon JH. Prevention of citrate intoxication during exchange transfusion. JAMA. 1963;183:163.
100. Huestis DW, Fletcher JL, White RF, et al. Citrate anticoagulants for plateletpheresis. Transfusion. 1977;17:151.
101. Olson PR, Cox C, McCullough J. Laboratory and clinical effects of the infusion of ACD solution during plateletpheresis. Vox Sang. 1977;33:79.
102. Mishler JM, Hadlock DC, Fortuny IE, et al. Increased efficiency of leukocyte collection by the addition of hydroxyethyl starch to the continuous flow centrifuge. Blood. 1974;44:571.
103. Alavi JB, Root RK, Djerassi I, et al. A randomized clinical trial of granulocyte transfusions for infection in acute leukemia. N Engl J Med. 1977;296:706.
104. Herzig RH, Herzig GP, Graw RG, et al. Successful granulocyte transfusion therapy for gram-negative septicemia: a prospectively randomized controlled study. N Engl J Med. 1977;296:701.

105. Walker EM, Cannon A, Mitchum EN. Current status of leukocyte and platelet administration in cancer therapy. Ann Clin Lab Sci. 1983;13:453.
106. Cooper MR. Indications for granulocyte transfusion. Prog Clin Biol Res. 1982;88:43.
107. Ford JM, Cullen MH, Roberts MM, et al. Prophylactic granulocyte transfusions: results of a randomized controlled trial in patients with acute myelogenous leukemia. Transfusion. 1982;22:311.
108. Christensen RD, Rothstein G, Anstall HB, et al. Granulocyte transfusions in neonates with bacterial infection, neutropenia and depletion of mature marrow neutrophils. Pediatrics. 1982;70:1.
109. Laurenti F, Ferro R, Isacchi G, et al. Polymorphonuclear leukocyte transfusion for the treatment of sepsis in the newborn infant. J Pediatr. 1981;98:118.
110. Siegel J, McCracken G. Sepsis neonatorum. N Engl J Med. 1981;304:642.
111. Christensen RD, Anstall HB, Rothstein G. Review: deficiencies in the neutrophil system of newborn infants, and the use of leukocyte transfusions in the treatment of neonatal sepsis. J Clin Apheresis. 1982;1:33.
112. Ring J, Seifert J, Messmer K, Brendal W. Anaphylactoid reactions due to hydroxyethyl starch infusion. Eur Surg Res. 1976;8:389.
113. Rock G, Wise P. Plasma expansion during granulocyte procurement: cumulative effects of hydroxyethyl starch. Blood. 1979;53:1156.
114. Bode U, Deisseroth AB. Donor toxicity in granulocyte collections: association of lichen planus with the use of hydroxyethyl starch leukapheresis. Transfusion. 1979;21:83.
115. Newman RS, Barr RJ, Ocariz JA, et al. Does hydroxyethyl starch cause lichen planus? Lichen planus in a long-time routine blood donor never exposed to hydroxyethyl starch. Transfusion. 1983;23:531.
116. Dahlke MB, Shah SL, Sherwood WC, et al. Priapism during filtration leukapheresis. Transfusion. 1979;19:482.
117. Leitman SF, Boltansky H, Alter HJ, et al. Allergic reactions in healthy plateletpheresis donors caused by sensitization to ethylene oxide gas. N Engl J Med. 1986;315:1192.
118. Grammer LC, Roberts M, Nicholls AJ, et al. IgE against ethylene oxide-altered human serum albumin in patients who have had acute dialysis reactions. J Allergy Clin Immunol. 1984;74:544.

# CHAPTER 2

# REDUCED COMPATIBILITY TESTING

## ABBREVIATED COMPATIBILITY TESTING

Containing the cost of medical care in the United States is one of the largest challenges facing the nation. Health care costs are becoming an increasingly larger percentage of the gross national product. Many changes in reimbursement plans to both hospitals and physicians have been put into place with the hopes that health care costs can be held steady or even reversed. Diagnostic-related groups (DRGs) are an example of such policies. A DRG mandates that a set dollar figure will be given to a hospital for reimbursement based on a patient's diagnosis regardless of the length of stay. This policy gives financial incentives to hospitals for short inpatient stays and reduces the number of diagnostic procedures. Hospital laboratories have been especially hard hit with financial cutbacks and the need to become more efficient.

Along with the demand to become fiscally sound are increased requirements from the Joint Commission on Accreditation of Healthcare Organizations (JCAHO) to improve patient care through quality assurance. Improved quality assurance programs should help control overall health care costs by improving the appropriate use of ancillary services. The laboratory is called on to monitor high-risk, problem-prone, and high-volume indicators, including the careful scrutiny of the use of blood products. Although these efforts are extremely important in assuring quality patient care, they nevertheless take time and financial resources at a time when laboratories are being asked to cut spending. This necessitates the careful evaluation of cost-to-benefit ratios for expenditure of laboratory personnel and resources.

The pretransfusion compatibility test is an area of laboratory medicine in which costs can be reduced. More importantly, limited compatibility testing protocols can make the management of a limited blood supply more efficient. Since blood can be released faster after request, fewer units need to be reserved per patient, which can reduce the inventory requirements of many blood banks. The compatibility test is composed of many parts and is not synonymous with a crossmatch. Shulman and

Kent[1] describe the compatibility test as including: 1) determining the ABO and Rh type of the donor blood; 2) detecting unexpected red blood cell (RBC) antibodies in the donor's plasma; 3) determining the ABO and Rh type of the patient from an accurately labeled specimen; 4) researching previous laboratory records and comparing with current laboratory records and results; 5) detecting unexpected RBC antibodies in the patient's plasma; and 6) matching ABO-compatible RBC products and performing major crossmatch, or equivalent test, to detect ABO incompatibility between the patient's serum and donor RBCs.

### The Immediate Spin Crossmatch

The antiglobulin test (AGT) phase of compatibility testing has been in place for many years and was designed to be extremely sensitive in detecting antibodies in a patient's serum that could cause overt hemolysis or shortened survival of donor RBCs after transfusion. Many blood group systems have been discovered after finding an antibody during the AGT phase of the crossmatch. In 1964, Grove-Rasmussen[2] demonstrated the efficacy of eliminating the AGT phase of the crossmatch, provided that a screening test is performed using an AGT and is found to be negative. Many authors have reported similar findings.[3-13] Different approaches to modifying compatibility testing exist, but most involve replacing the AGT phase of a major crossmatch with an immediate spin crossmatch (ISXM). The purpose of the ISXM is to check for ABO incompatibility prior to release of RBCs. Advantages of the ISXM over the AGT crossmatch include the following: 1) blood can be released faster during clinically urgent situations; 2) the quicker release time allows for the reservation of fewer units per patient, making more blood available to the general blood inventory; 3) technologist time can be focused more on the prevention of clerical errors; and 4) reagent costs can be reduced.

In 1981, Garratty[6] reviewed studies that included nearly 1 million crossmatches and showed that the risk of missing a "clinically significant" antibody using an antibody screen, in place of an AGT crossmatch, was 1 in 17,000 crossmatches. In the 11th edition of AABB *Standards for Blood Banks and Transfusion Services*,[14] the requirement for the AGT phase of the crossmatch was dropped if no unexpected antibodies are found during the screening procedure, which must include an AGT. While most regulatory agencies have dropped the requirement for the AGT phase of the crossmatch, surveys estimate that only 11% of the hospitals in the United States have replaced the AGT phase of the crossmatch with an ISXM or equivalent method testing for ABO incompatibility. The reason behind this small percentage of hospitals using the ISXM instead of an AGT crossmatch is not entirely clear, but some of the limitations of the ISXM will be discussed.

Unlike the minor crossmatch, which has been shown not to make transfusion of blood safer to the patient, the AGT phase of compatibility testing does provide an added level of safety. Transfusion services must consider various factors when deciding to implement the ISXM. The ISXM is used to detect ABO incompatibility for patients with a negative antibody screen and lacking a history of RBC alloantibodies. The antibody screen becomes the primary method for detecting unexpected antibodies in the patient's serum when using an ISXM. Reports of the failure of a screening procedure to detect clinically significant antibodies exist.[1-13, 15-21] To minimize these failures, attention must be given to the number of screening cells used, the spectrum of antigens covered by these screening cells, and the dosage of various antigens present on the screening cells. The screen can also be made more sensitive for certain antigens by including an enzyme technique.

The sensitivity of the ISXM for detecting ABO incompatibility is generally reported to be between 99% and 100%,[7] but the sensitivity can drop to approximately 50% in $A_2B$ donor cells crossmatched with B serum.[8,17,18] The ISXM can also give false-negative results secondary to the prozone phenomenon with high anti-A and/or anti-B titers.[16] This problem seems to occur secondary to the steric hindrance of hemagglutination by the C1 component of complement. This cause of a false-negative ISXM can be removed by using reagents containing ethylenediaminetetraacetic acid (EDTA), which will bind calcium needed for the assembly of C1 subunits.

Failure of a screening procedure in combination with an ISXM to detect a "clinically significant" antibody does not always result in a hemolytic transfusion reaction. A recent survey[9] examined 1.3 million crossmatches and found 5 cases of overt in vivo hemolysis caused by antibodies missed during the screen and ISXM procedures. Each of these antibodies was detected during the transfusion reaction work-up where an AGT crossmatch was performed. None of the cases were complicated by disseminated intravascular coagulation, renal failure, or death. The calculated rate of overt hemolytic reaction per ISXM was 1 in 250,000. The author appropriately concluded that the decision to use an ISXM procedure must be made by individual blood banks, and the published rates of overt hemolytic reactions using an ISXM will be viewed positively by some institutions and negatively by others.

If the use of an ISXM is contemplated, a strategy must be employed for dealing with false-positive results. Most false-positive ISXMs are caused by rouleaux or cold-reacting antibodies. Technologists must be able to distinguish true ABO incompatibility from false-positive reactions to prevent unnecessary delays in issuing blood, which could compromise patient care.

The ISXM is used as a safeguard to prevent the transfusion of an ABO-incompatible unit of RBCs. Some authors have argued that instead of performing a major crossmatch, time would be better spent on retyping of the patient and donor unit, as well as having 2 people check labels and paperwork at the time blood is issued.[19,20] Studies have demonstrated the efficacy of eliminating the major crossmatch if another protocol is used to prevent ABO incompatibility.[1,7] Small clerical error rates were observed with the elimination of the major crossmatch, and differences were observed between a noncrossmatch protocol used in an ideal working environment compared to a busy blood bank. It was believed that this small error rate can be eliminated with the use of a laboratory information system that alerts technologists to ABO incompatibility between patient and donor.

### Value of the Autocontrol

The autocontrol is another part of pretransfusion testing that has come under scrutiny.[10,21,22] The autocontrol is valuable when the eluate from the patient's own cells leads to the identification of an antibody that could shorten RBC survival but is not yet detectable in the antibody screen. The rates of significant antibodies detected from autocontrol-positive/antibody screen–negative samples range from 1 in 14,548 to 25 in 56,090. It is not surprising that various groups have decided to retain or delete the autocontrol from pretransfusion testing based on the efficiency of the autocontrol in their particular laboratory.

Decisions to abbreviate pretransfusion testing, whether the AGT crossmatch, the autocontrol, or both (by replacement with another method to determine ABO incompatibility), should not be made until parallel testing has been performed in the laboratory contemplating a change.

## References


1. Shulman IA, Kent D. Safety in transfusion practice. Arch Pathol Lab Med. 1989;113:270.
2. Grove-Rasmussen M. Routine compatibility testing. Transfusion. 1964;4:200.
3. Shulman IA, Nelson JM, Kent DR, et al. Experience with a cost-effective crossmatch protocol. JAMA. 1985;254:93.
4. Oberman HA, Barnes BA, Friedman BA. The risk of abbreviating the major crossmatch in urgent or massive transfusion. Transfusion. 1978;18:137.
5. Shulman IA, Nelson JM, Saxena S, et al. Experience with the routine use of an abbreviated crossmatch. Am J Clin Pathol. 1984;82:178.
6. Garratty G. The role of compatibility tests. Transfusion. 1982;22:169.
7. Meyer EA, Shulman IA. The sensitivity and specificity of the immediate-spin crossmatch. Transfusion. 1989;29:99.
8. Berry-Dortch S, Woodside CH, Boral LI. Limitation of the immediate spin crossmatch when used for detecting ABO incompatibility. Transfusion. 1985;25:176.
9. Shulman IA. The risk of an overt hemolytic transfusion reaction following the use of an immediate spin crossmatch. Arch Pathol Lab Med. 1990;114:412.

10. Perkins JT, Arruza M, Fong K, et al. The relative utility of the autologous control and the antiglobulin phase of the crossmatch. Transfusion. 1990;30:503.
11. Boral LI, Henry JB. The type and screen: a safe alternative and supplement in selected surgical procedures. Transfusion. 1977;17:163.
12. Oberman HA, Barnes BA, Steiner EA. Role of the crossmatch in testing for serologic incompatibility. Transfusion. 1982;22:12.
13. Heisto H. Pretransfusion blood group serology: limited value of the antiglobulin phase of the crossmatch when a careful screening test for unexpected antibodies is performed. Transfusion. 1979;19:761.
14. Schmidt PJ, ed. Standards for Blood Banks and Transfusion Services. 11th ed. Arlington, Va: American Association of Blood Banks; 1984:25.
15. Mitten EA, Gregory KR, Schmidt PJ. Double failure of the type and screen. Am J Clin Pathol. 1987;87:252.
16. Judd WJ, Steiner EA, O'Donnell DB, et al. Discrepancies in reverse ABO typing due to prozone: how safe is the immediate-spin crossmatch? Transfusion. 1988;28:334.
17. Shulman IA, Nelson JM, Lam HT, et al. Unreliability of the immediate-spin cross-match to detect ABO incompatibility (letter). Transfusion. 1985;25:589.
18. Shulman IA, Nelson JM, Lam HT, et al. Additional limitations of the immediate-spin crossmatch to detect ABO incompatibility (letter). Am J Clin Pathol. 1987;87:677.
19. Hafleigh EB. Cited in: Garratty G. The role of compatibility tests. Transfusion. 1982;22:169.
20. Svoboda R. Passing the crossmatch by screening antibodies. Lab World. 1981;32:26.
21. Judd WJ, Barnes EA, Steiner HA, et al. The evaluation of a positive direct antiglobulin test (autocontrol) in pretransfusion testing revisited. Transfusion. 1986;26:220.
22. Huh YO, Lichtiger B. Evaluation of a autologous control in pretransfusion testing. Am J Clin Pathol. 1985;84:632.

## CHAPTER 3

# TRANSFUSION-TRANSMISSIBLE DISEASES

## INFECTIOUS HEPATITIS

Blood and blood products may be infectious. Viral, bacterial, and parasitic diseases have been transmitted by the parenteral administration of blood. One of the most serious diseases transmitted is viral hepatitis.

Infectious hepatitis is not a new disease. The Chinese described accounts of contagious jaundice millennia ago.[1] Five centuries before Christ, the Babylonian Talmud described jaundice with other liver diseases.[2,3] In this same period, Hippocrates described contagious or epidemic jaundice as 1 of the 4 kinds of jaundice. During times of war, the disruption of society leads to dislocation of people, inadequate sewage disposal, and contamination of food and drinking water. Hepatitis or "campaign jaundice" frequently afflicted soldiers, and epidemic jaundice among civilians was often seen.[4]

A second type of infectious hepatitis has been recognized. This form of hepatitis is transmitted by the transfusion of blood or administration of blood products. Patients who have received red blood cell transfusion for anemia or plasma products for protection against smallpox, measles, mumps, or yellow fever have subsequently developed jaundice.[3,5] This form of hepatitis has been called "serum hepatitis" to distinguish it from the epidemic or "infectious hepatitis."

In the 1940s, the clinical features of "infectious hepatitis" and "serum hepatitis" began to be clarified.[6] Studies with volunteers demonstrated that the 2 were distinct entities. Epidemic jaundice or infectious hepatitis was usually acquired by the ingestion of fecally contaminated food or water. The disease typically occurred in families or groups of individuals. Infectious hepatitis had a short incubation period, 15 to 33 days. In contrast, serum hepatitis followed exposure to blood products and had an incubation period of 50 to 60 days. Prior exposure to one form of hepatitis did not confer immunity to the second. Because of the differences in the clinical course and epidemiology, the terminology of hepatitis A for infectious hepatitis and hepatitis B for serum hepatitis was adopted.

The development of serum transaminase assays to measure liver injury in the 1950s further separated these 2 forms of hepatitis.[7] Patients with serum hepatitis had prolonged periods of abnormal transaminase activity, 35 to 200 days. Those with infectious hepatitis had briefer periods of increased serum enzyme activity.

Differentiation of hepatitis A and hepatitis B by serologic methods followed. An antigen was detected in the serum of an Australian patient with leukemia, who had been transfused.[8] The Australian antigen was also detected in the blood of transfused patients during the incubation period for serum hepatitis.[9] This antigen has been proved to be a component of the hepatitis B virus (HBV).[10] Extensive investigation of the virus has been made. The HBV genome has been sequenced and the molecular biology well described.[11]

The virus responsible for hepatitis A (HAV) has also been detected.[12] Specific serologic tests were developed for infectious hepatitis.[13] The HAV genome has been cloned and characterized,[14] and the viral proteins have been isolated and studied.[15]

## Hepatitis A

In contrast to hepatitis B virus, which is well recognized as a cause of posttransfusion hepatitis, hepatitis A virus has rarely caused hepatitis following blood transfusion.[16] However, because incidences of transfusion-related disease have been described,[17-19] and to further distinguish hepatitis A from other forms of posttransfusion hepatitis, the virus and the disease it causes merit discussion.

### Biologic Characteristics

The hepatitis A virus is a ribonucleic acid (RNA) virus in the family Picornaviridae and subgroup enterovirus, designated enterovirus 72.[20] The enteroviruses include the polioviruses, coxsackieviruses, and echoviruses. These viruses inhabit the human alimentary tract and may cause disease. Infection with the poliovirus and coxsackievirus causes human myelitis, paralysis, aseptic meningitis, encephalitis, respiratory illness, and other diseases. Echovirus infection similarly has caused meningitis, paralysis, encephalitis, and respiratory illnesses. Infection with hepatitis A virus causes liver disease.[21]

The hepatitis A virus genome is single-stranded RNA, approximately 7500 nucleotides in length. The RNA acts as messenger RNA (mRNA) in the cytoplasm of host cells, and it translates into a single protein strand. The protein undergoes proteolytic cleavage to form the viral structural proteins and the viral proteins for replication. The hepatitis A virus virion has 3 major structural proteins: VP1, VP2, and VP3. These are 22,000 to 33,000 d in size. A fourth smaller structural protein, VP4, is also present. In addition to these 4, there are other nonstructural replicative proteins, such as the RNA-dependent RNA polymerase.[22]

The HAV is small, 27 to 32 nm in size, roughly spherical with icosahedral symmetry. Its buoyant density is 1.33 g/mL[3] in cesium chloride and the sedimentation coefficient is 156s.[23] The virus lacks a lipoprotein capsule. Like other members of the enterovirus genus (ie, poliovirus, coxsackievirus, and echovirus), HAV is resistant to acid and probably replicates in the gastrointestinal tract. Hepatitis A virus differs from other members of the picornavirus family and enterovirus genus by surviving heat inactivation to 60°C.[22] In addition, nucleic acid and amino acid sequencing of HAV shows little homology with the other picornaviruses. Although its molecular structure is similar to members of its genus, it is only distantly related to enterovirus at the level of nucleotide and protein sequencing.

The virus replicates in the cytoplasm of infected cells. The RNA serves as a template for negative-stranded RNA, which in turn is used to form additional viral RNA or mRNA. The mechanism of picornaviral replication has been characterized.[24]

Hepatitis A virus has been cultured in primate cells where it causes no cytopathic effects. Routine culture is not useful as a diagnostic technique because the wild virus grows poorly in cell culture. With passage of the virus in cultured cells, an adapted virus is formed that grows better in culture. This virus causes persistent infection in cell culture, in contrast to the near absence of chronic persistent HAV infections in vivo.[25]

### Identification and Serology

The virus is shed in the stools of the infected.[12] The virus may be identified in the feces by immunologic methods. The techniques most commonly used are enzyme immunoassay (EIA), radioimmunoassay (RIA), and immune electron microscopy (IEM).[22] Viral antigen detection in stool specimens is not a useful clinical test. By the time a patient seeks medical attention because of the symptoms, the peak gastrointestinal shedding of HAV has passed.

Serologic identification of antibodies to HAV are more useful in clinical settings. The HAV has been found to have a single antigenicity, and serum antibody has usually been formed during the incubation period. For the specific diagnosis of HAV acute infection, IgM class-specific antibody assays have been developed. The specific IgM response is short-lived, 2 to 12 months. Assays are usually positive within a week of the illness and usually negative by 6 months.[20] A total serologic titer is not helpful in the diagnosis of acute hepatitis A, because about 50% of American adults have had prior exposure to HAV. In addition, acute and convalescent sera often show little difference in total antibody titer.[22] IgG levels of anti-HAV persist for many years to the lifetime of the patient.

### Typical Disease in the Nontransfused Individual

Exposure to HAV often follows ingestion of fecally contaminated food or water. Outbreaks of hepatitis A within a community have been traced to a single source. The sources have included water, shellfish harvested in waters contaminated by sewage, and food prepared by food handlers infected with the virus.[20] However, these common-source food or water-borne outbreaks account for 10% of patients with hepatitis A (Figure 3-1). Contact with a person who has hepatitis A can be found in about 30% of infected patients.[26] Person-to-person contact with children in day-care centers accounts for another 12% to 16% of patients with the disease.

**FIGURE 3-1** Exposure history of individuals with hepatitis A. In the majority of cases, a specific source cannot be identified.

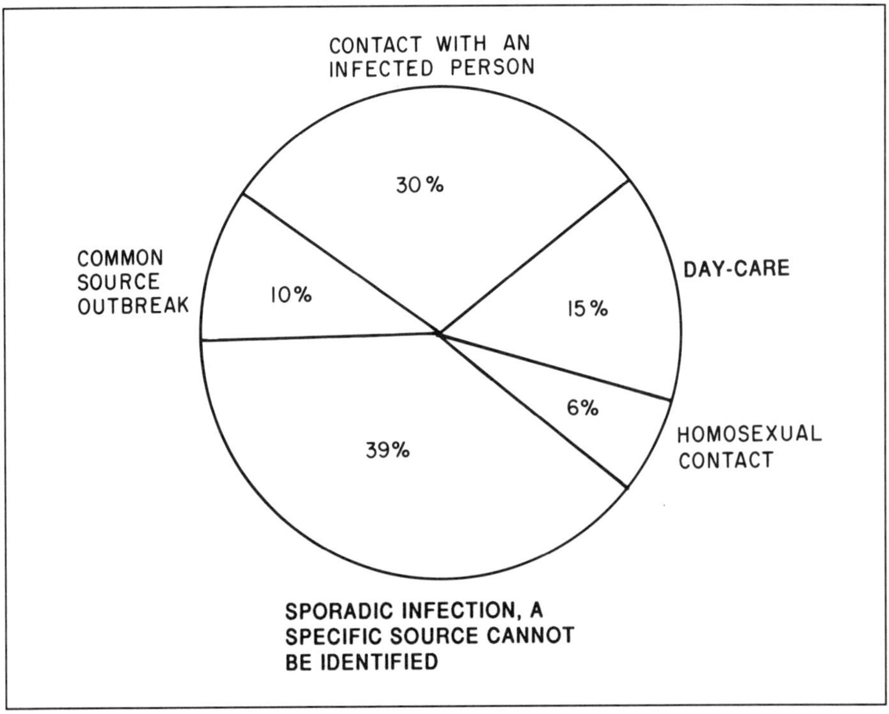

Outbreaks in day-care centers are more common in those centers that enroll younger children still in diapers.[27] A history of homosexual contact can be elicited in another 6% of patients with hepatitis A, and acquisition of the virus has been correlated with oral-anal sexual contact.[28] The disease occurs sporadically in the remaining patients, and a specific source for the infection cannot be identified.

The average incubation period from exposure to HAV to symptomatic disease is 30 days (Figure 3-2), with a range of 15 to 45 days. This is the incubation period observed clinically and verified experimentally.[7] The relatively short incubation period of HAV contrasts with the longer, 70-day average, incubation time for HBV.[29]

The disease of acute viral hepatitis caused by HAV is clinically similar to the hepatitis due to HBV. The initial symptoms are nonspecific and may include malaise, weakness, anorexia, nausea, and vomiting. Right

**FIGURE 3-2** Following exposure to HAV, the virus is shed in the stool and circulates in blood before the onset of symptoms. Antibody to the virus begins to be produced while the patient is symptomatic.

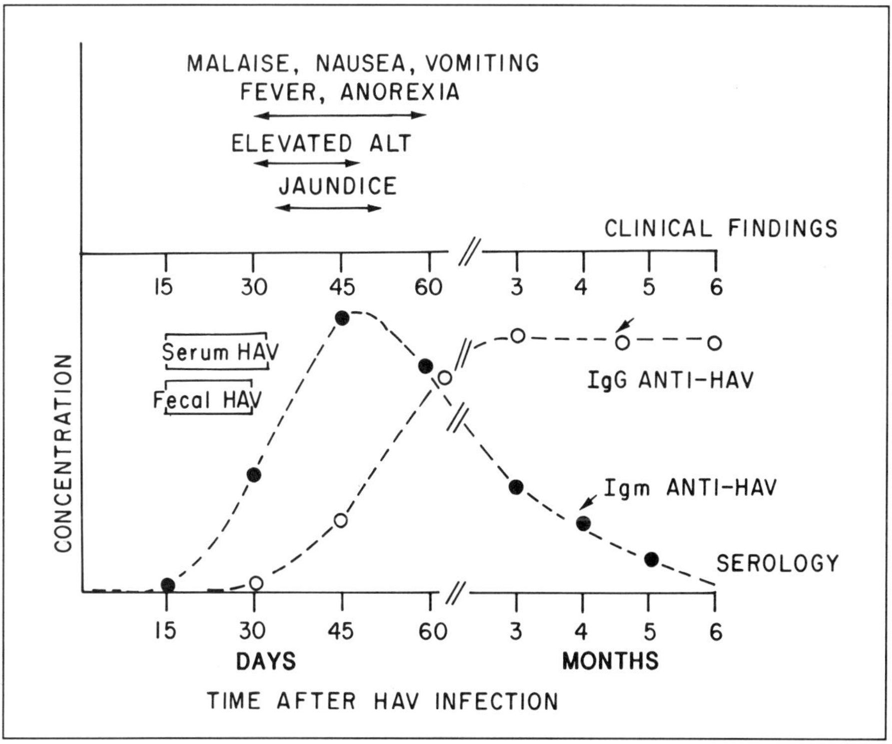

upper quadrant abdominal pain is sometimes present.[23] These symptoms precede by days the development of jaundice and dark urine (Figure 3-2). The duration of these signs and symptoms in hepatitis A infection is generally less than 60 days, and the disease is self-limited. Occasionally a patient has prolonged jaundice for several months, but this resolves as well.[30] Some patients also have symptomatic exacerbations or relapses.

Fulminant hepatitis or massive hepatic necrosis from the HAV is unusual, occurring in far less than 1% of infections.[10] Patients present with signs and symptoms of encephalopathy. There are disturbances in consciousness and behavior. Focal and generalized neurologic signs are present, including rigidity, hyperreflexia, and seizures. Electroencephalograms (EEGs) may be abnormal. Elevated serum ammonia levels support the diagnosis of hepatic encephalopathy.[31] Fulminant hepatitis is also associated with a markedly elevated serum bilirubin and a prolonged prothrombin time. The liver shrinks in size. Other complications of massive hepatic necrosis include cerebral edema, gastrointestinal bleeding, sepsis, cardiovascular collapse, respiratory failure, and renal failure. Fulminant and fatal hepatic necrosis is seen in less than 1% of patients hospitalized with hepatitis A.[23]

In contrast to the infrequent occurrence of fulminant disease, cases of asymptomatic infection with HAV are common.[32] More than 80% of children younger than 2 years of age and infected with HAV are asymptomatic. The percentage of persons with asymptomatic infection decreases with age. Of healthy adolescents in the United States, 19% have serologic evidence of prior hepatitis A without a history of clinical disease. Adults have the lowest incidence of asymptomatic infection; only slightly more than 10% of infected adults have no symptoms.[32]

Laboratory studies assist the diagnosis of acute viral hepatitis. The hepatic enzymes, serum aspartate aminotransferase (AST) and alanine aminotransferase (ALT), may be increased from 5 to more than 100 times normal. The alkaline phosphatase (Alk P), another hepatic enzyme, is only mildly elevated. The hepatic enzyme levels become abnormal during the late incubation period, before the onset of jaundice. With jaundice, the serum bilirubin is elevated with nearly equal increases of conjugated (direct) and nonconjugated (indirect) bilirubin. The ALT level remains abnormal in symptomatic patients, the elevated serum enzyme levels persist for several weeks after the icterus, and the hyperbilirubinemia resolves.[22]

Infection with hepatitis A is accompanied by a polyclonal hyperglobulinemia, with an early increase in IgM.[33-35] Antibodies to HAV, anti-HAV, can be directly measured. The rise in IgM antibody titers precedes the development of jaundice. The detection of anti-HAV IgM level correlates with recent infections, and the serum levels of IgM anti-HAV persist for 6 to 12 months. Serum IgG anti-HAV titers persist for longer periods after the infection. An elevated IgG level indicates previous exposure to HAV. Epidemiologists have used the detection of IgG anti-HAV to determine the prevalence of HAV in the communities they have studied.

The virus is shed in the feces of infected patients.[12] The peak amount of virus release precedes the symptomatic phase. A person incubating the virus may be spreading the disease unaware of the contagious risk. Within households the infectious risk to susceptible contacts is 70% to 83%.[36]

Direct culture of the virus from stool is difficult, because the wild-type virus grows poorly in cell culture.[25] However, the diagnosis may be made by the extraction of viral RNA from the feces followed by molecular hybridization with clone HAV cDNA[37] or demonstration of the HAV antigen by immunologic techniques.[12] These techniques are not used in routine clinical settings.

Brief periods of viremia have been demonstrated by the infectivity of serum administered experimentally by mouth or by intramuscular injection.[7] Levels of virus in both serum and feces decline after antibodies develop, and chronic hepatic virus production does not occur with HAV.[23]

The prevalence of the disease has been estimated in epidemiologic investigations by total anti-HAV levels. Two different epidemiologic patterns have been seen in different parts of the world.[22] In the first pattern, seen in most parts of the world, the prevalence of anti-HAV is 100% before the teenage years. In most of the world, infection with HAV is similar to other enteric diseases, occurring as a disease, often asymptomatic, of childhood. The epidemiologic investigations have shown that exposure to the virus is usually not associated with symptomatic hepatitis; a history of jaundice is not elicited from every person with antibody. Children with clinically apparent hepatitis A have only mild or nonspecific symptoms, without the development of jaundice.[7,26]

The second pattern is seen in more developed countries Childhood infection is less common, and the incidence of adult exposure increases with age. Infection with HAV later in life is more frequently symptomatic than infection in childhood. In these countries sporadic cases or epidemics may occur following a breakdown of sanitary barriers. In this setting, HAV becomes a major public health problem.[22] The administration of pooled immune serum globulin provides protection from hepatitis A.

To summarize, HAV is typically acquired following the fecal contamination of food or water. In the less developed countries, exposure occurs in childhood, and the infection is often asymptomatic. Disease in adults is more severe, but self-limited, and death is rare. The virus is shed in the feces only during the incubation phase of infection, and viremia occurs. The infection is self-limited, and no chronic carrier state is seen.

### Typical Disease in the Transfused Individual

Hepatitis A virus is a rare cause of transfusion-associated hepatitis. A review of thousands of cases of posttransfusion hepatitis failed to identify any caused by HAV.[38] However, infection with HAV has been described in a limited number of transfusion-associated diseases. Donor blood may be infected with HAV if the unit is drawn during the viremic phase of the disease.[7] Viremia occurs in the incubation period, before symptoms of illness occur in the donor.

Only a few reports of posttransfusion hepatitis A have been described. In 1981, Seeberg and colleagues[17] from Sweden reported that 3 nurses in a pediatric surgery ward developed jaundice, and epidemic hepatitis was suspected. Six other staff members became ill, and a child on the ward also developed jaundice. Epidemiologic investigation identified a mother and child as the likely index cases. The mother had signs of hepatitis, and the baby's serum had anti-HAV IgM. The baby had previously had an exchange blood transfusion for neonatal jaundice. The blood donor was a man who had traveled in an endemic area. He was well when he donated blood but 10 days later developed signs of hepatitis, and hepatitis A was diagnosed serologically.

The other reports are similar, describing hepatitis A occurring in a patient who received blood from an initially asymptomatic donor who then developed jaundice. In 1 report, the blood recipient developed jaundice 3 weeks after transfusion, and serologic studies confirmed hepatitis A.[39] In another case, the blood donor developed fulminant fatal hepatitis A. The donated unit had been transfused into a young girl who developed icteric jaundice. Hepatitis A antigen was identified in the donor unit, and inoculation of donor plasma into a chimpanzee resulted in development of hepatitis A in the animal.[18] Another report[19] details how a single unit of HAV-infected blood was transfused into 11 neonates. Newborns, nurses, physicians, and family members became infected. Serologic studies confirmed the presence of anti-HAV IgM in the neonates, and symptomatic hepatitis was diagnosed in the adult hospital staff and family members. The infants who received the blood were asymptomatic, but they passed the infection to the adults caring for them. None of the transfused neonates died or developed chronic liver disease.

### Steps Taken to Minimize the Risks

Because of the extremely small risk of acquiring hepatitis A from transfusion, and the typically mild and self-limited nature of the infection, studies for the HAV antigen or antibodies are not routinely performed on donor blood. The screening questions for prospective donors attempt to exclude those who may be incubating HAV. Individuals who have had prior contact with jaundiced individuals, who have recently traveled out of the country, or who have been exposed to any infections are asked not to donate.

Another factor that limits the potential infectivity of donor blood is the early rise of anti-HAV IgM, usually preceding the onset of jaundice.[23]

Because pooled immunoglobulin may be administered to protect against short-term exposure to hepatitis A,[40] it is likely that the donor's antibody reduces the risk of infection in the blood recipient.

### Infectivity of Blood Products

The rare reports of HAV infection are limited to transfusion of blood. No reports describe infection from plasma or other products.

## Hepatitis B

Jaundice following the percutaneous administration of blood, blood products, or serum has been recognized for more than 100 years. In retrospect, the first recorded epidemic of hepatitis B probably occurred in Germany in the 1830s. A group of 1289 shipyard workers received a smallpox vaccine made from human lymphatic fluid. Weeks to months later, 15% of those inoculated with the vaccine developed jaundice.[5] In 1937, another epidemic was seen. A group of 109 children were inoculated with human convalescent plasma for passive protection against measles. Later, 41 of the children developed jaundice. In 1942, an epidemic occurred in 28,585 members of the U.S. Armed Forces. The Armed Forces members were vaccinated prophylactically for yellow fever, a flavivirus disease spread by mosquitoes. The hepatitis was transmitted by batches of the vaccine that had been contaminated by hepatitis B virus.[41] In 1943, infectious jaundice was described following the transfusion of blood products rather than prophylactic vaccination.[41]

Hepatitis has been spread by the use of contaminated needles and syringes.[42] In the past, individuals treated at 1 clinic with parenteral arsenic for syphilis developed hepatitis B. An investigation of treatment techniques at the clinic revealed that syringes used for multiple inoculations had spread the disease.[42] Undoubtedly, many of these jaundice and hepatitis cases were due to HBV.

In the 1940s and 1950s, experimental transmission studies defined differences between infectious or epidemic hepatitis and serum hepatitis. The diseases differed in their incubation periods, and there was a complete lack of cross-immunity for the 2 forms of hepatitis.[6,7] Unfortunately in the 1960s, serum hepatitis from the transfusion of blood occurred in as many as 22% of patients receiving blood.[43] Hepatitis B surface antigen (HBsAg) was identified in serum of a transfused patient with leukemia in 1965 by Blumberg and associates, and it has provided the blood banks with a marker of HBV infection.[8,9] The ability to screen blood products for HBsAg has reduced the incidence of posttransfusion infection due to HBV.[44] Even with serologic screening, however, posttransfusion HBV infections have continued to occur.[49] When sought, HBV DNA has been identified in 2% of blood donors who are negative for the usual HBV markers or elevated transaminases.[46] Hepatitis B virus remains an important infective agent for posttransfusion hepatitis.

**Biologic Characteristics**

Hepatitis B virus is a small enveloped DNA virus, 42 nm in diameter, with a tropism for hepatocytes.[11] The hepatitis B virus has properties that distinguish it from other DNA viruses. HBV belongs to the hepaDNA virus family, which includes other hepatic HBV-like viruses found in animals.

The HBV genome is a circular, partially double-stranded DNA molecule (Figure 3-3). Complete nucleotide sequences have been determined for several of the different HBV subtypes. The long strand of DNA has a fixed length of about 3200 nucleotides and is not quite a closed circle. This is the DNA minus strand, which has the protein coding capacity of the virus. The short, incomplete DNA plus strand is of variable length from 15% to 65% of the circumference of the minus strand. The plus strand maintains the circular structure of the DNA by base pairing with the minus strand at the two 5' ends.

The HBV replicates in the nuclei of hepatocytes. The DNA replication involves an unusual reverse transcriptase step in which HBV RNA is made and then copied back into DNA plus strand.[11] Viral DNA polymerase is complexed with the three feet end of the plus strand to begin the additional DNA synthesis steps.

Proteins are encoded by the minus viral DNA strand, including both structural proteins and enzymes. The virion carries a DNA-dependent DNA polymerase in the viral core.[11] The HBV DNA has been cloned in bacterial cells, and from these[47] the complete nucleotide sequence has been identified. The genetic map of HBV DNA is known.

The surface of the viral envelope is complex, and a variety of HBsAg subtypes may be formed.[48] The protein components of the envelope are coded by the S region of the gene. The viral core is antigenic for anti-HBcAg. The HBcAg is not found free in blood but is only contained in the viral envelope of the intact virion.

The virus is enclosed in a nucleocapsid, which is an electron-dense, 27 nm in diameter hexagon (Figure 3-3). The nucleocapsid is further encapsulated in a lipoprotein coat or viral envelope, 7 nm in width. This viral envelope is formed by membrane lipids and proteins that have the antigenicity of hepatitis B surface antigen (HBsAg). This complete virion is called a Dane particle. The hepatitis B virion has a spherical shape with a diameter of about 42 nm. Incomplete viral envelopes without DNA but with antigenicity of HBsAg are also present in large numbers in the serum of HBV-infected patients, consisting predominantly of 20 nm in diameter spherical particles.[11] Virus production continues for about 6 months in most adults. These HBsAg particles induce a protective antibody response to neutralize the virus in most infected individuals. Some patients have prolonged viral production and are designated as chronic HBsAg carriers.

The HBV has a host range restricted to humans and some other primates.[11] The virus may be infective by inoculation through the skin or mucous membranes. Some studies show infectivity following oral ingestion.[6] Hepatocytes are the main site of HBV infection, but viral DNA has also been found in the pancreas and in leukocytes.[11] The assembly with viral protein occurs in the cytoplasm.

## Serology

The first serologic marker of hepatitis B was an antigen identified in 1965 and called the Australia antigen.[9] The antigen currently is called the hepatitis B surface antigen (HBsAg). The surface antigen of HBV is complex, and 5 different antigenic specificities may be found.[48] The virus has a group-specific determinant, termed a. Two pairs of subtype antigens, or variants, are termed dy and wr. The subtypes usually behave as alleles, and serotypes have d or y and either r or w.

**FIGURE 3-3** Hepatitis B virus is a DNA virus with partially double-stranded DNA molecules. The viral genome is enclosed in a nucleocapsid and an envelope.

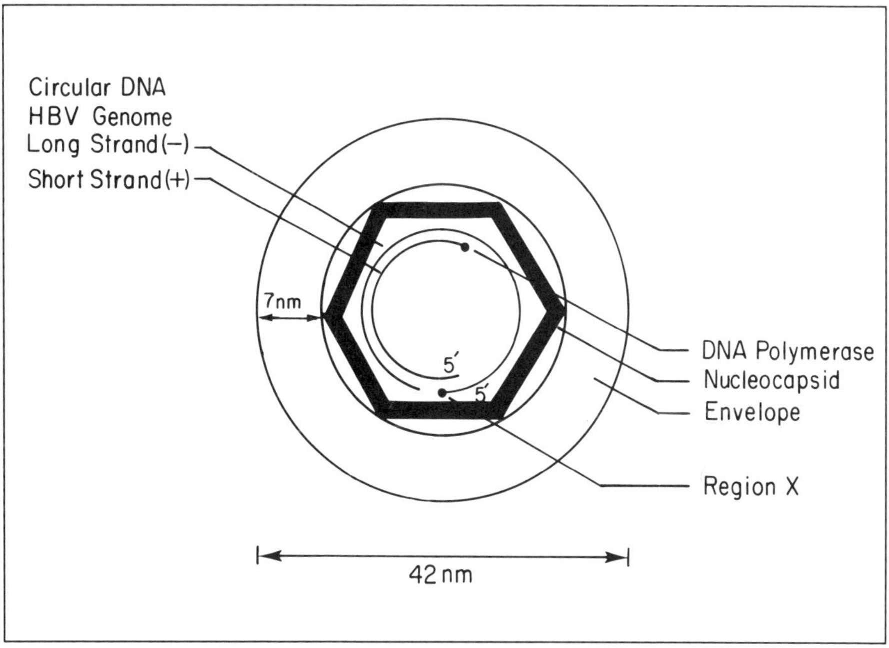

The HBsAg may be adr, adw, ayr, or ayw. These different subtypes predominate in different regions of the world and are useful in epidemiologic studies. Additional antigenic variants have been described: the w antigen determinant is heterogenic, and additional variants q, x, and g have been described.

The HBsAg is associated with the complete virion isolated from serum described by Dane and associates[49] (Figure 3-3). The virion is 42 nm in diameter with a 7-nm thick, lipid-containing outer envelope. The spherical inner core or nucleocapsid is 28 nm in diameter. Additional particles with surface antigen also circulate in plasma. Small spherical particles with diameters of 16 to 25 nm and rod-shaped forms 22 nm in width and up to hundreds of nm in length have been observed. These 2 antigenic forms contain protein, carbohydrate, and lipid, without nucleic acid or complete viral envelope. For every intact virus in circulation, hundreds of empty-coat particles are in circulation.[11]

The outer envelope of the HBV virion can be removed by treatment with detergents (Figure 3-4). This treatment frees core particles with HBV core antigen, HBcAg, which is distinct from HBsAg and does not circulate. The core also contains the viral DNA and associated viral protein. A cleavage product of the core structural protein is released when the virion cores are disrupted. This polypeptide is an additional HBV antigen, e antigen or HBeAg. This antigen may be found free in circulation. In most patients HBeAg is identified early in the course of the infection; it is cleared from plasma more rapidly than HBsAg. The host manufactures antibody to these 3 antigens: anti-HBs, anti-HBc, and anti-HBe.[48]

## Typical Disease in the Nontransfused Individual

Most individuals with clinically apparent hepatitis B infections have self-limited disease that resolves completely. Serologic testing has shown that many more individuals have had self-limited and subclinical disease that is diagnosed only in retrospect. In another subset of patients with HBV, the virus is expressed for long periods of time and the patients remain both infected and infectious.

### *Self-Limited Infections*

Infectious rates for HBV vary widely throughout the world. The carrier rate for the antigen HBsAg varies from less than 1% in North America to 8% to 15% in Africa and Southeast Asia.[20] Many more individuals have been infected in these populations, since the majority of infected persons with self-limited infections develop anti-HBV and clear HBsAg from plasma. In the high prevalence areas, a vertical route of transmission occurs from infected mothers to infants. Hepatitis B virus infections are also acquired later in childhood by nonpercutaneous exposure or by ill-defined percutaneous methods.

In low endemic areas, including North America, Western Europe, and Australia, neonatal and childhood infections are rare. Most infections occur in individuals in their early adult years.[20] Many of the hepatitis B infections in the United States are acquired by percutaneous routes[50] (Figure 3-5). Intravenous drug users are at high risk for exposure, as are homosexual men. The disease has also been transmitted by heterosexual contact. The HBV is found in semen and saliva, making the venereal transmission possible. Health care workers are also at risk. In many of the individuals with hepatitis B infections, a specific route of infection cannot be demonstrated.[50]

The incubation period from exposure to HBV to development of elevated serum transaminase levels is 41 to 110 days. This is longer than the 30- to 38-day incubation of hepatitis A.[6] Serologic studies show viral

**FIGURE 3-4** | Hepatitis B virus antigens are associated with different parts of virion: HBsAg is associated with the HBV envelope; HBcAg is associated with the viral core and nucleocapsid; HBeAg is associated with viral DNA and proteins.

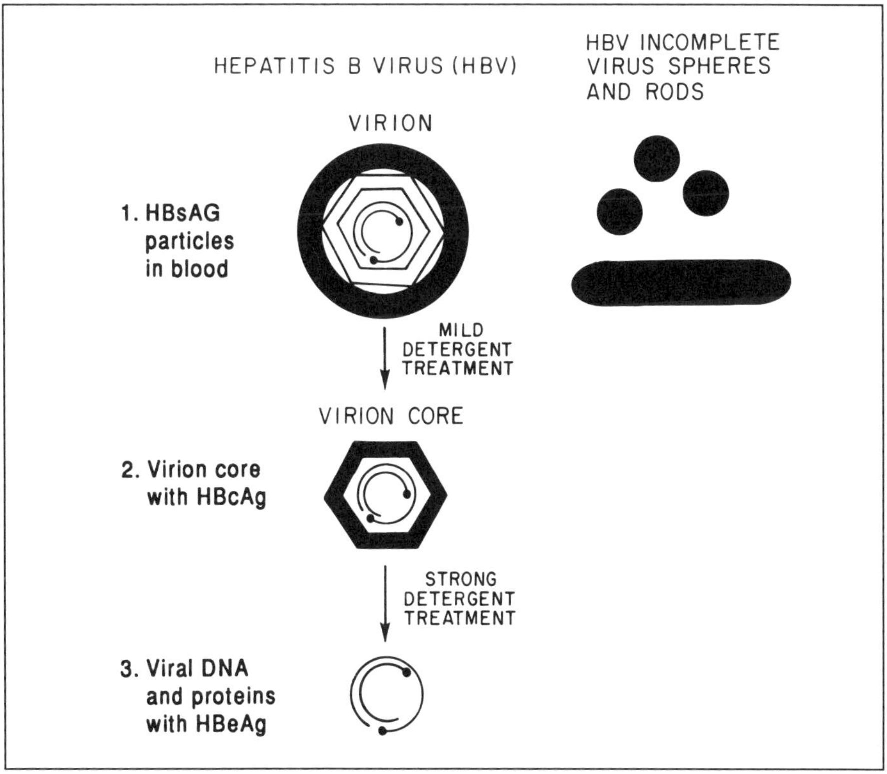

**Figure 3-5** | Exposure history of individuals infected with HBV.

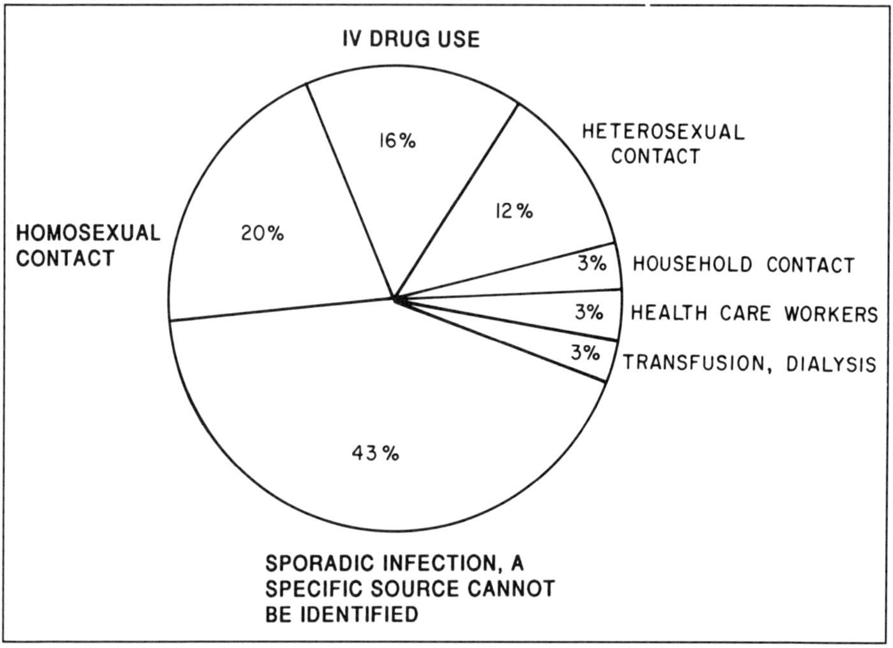


antigens HBsAg and HBeAg may appear in the blood as early as 7 days after the initial exposure to the virus[51] (Figure 3-6). The HBV antigens are present on average 4 weeks (range, 1–7 weeks) before clinical hepatitis is present.[51] In patients with self-limited hepatitis B infections, the HBsAg becomes negative 1 to 6 weeks after detection.

The prodromal symptoms seen clinically in viral hepatitis B are systemic. Patients have anorexia, nausea and vomiting, malaise, headache, myalgias, pharyngitis, and cough that precede the onset of jaundice by 7 to 14 days.[51] Dark urine and clay-colored stools also may be present before the onset of jaundice. Liver enlargement and tenderness are seen. During the recovery phase, constitutional symptoms abate. Serum transaminase levels rise before the onset of jaundice and return to normal after 3 to 4 months in patients with uncomplicated cases of hepatitis B infections.

Fatalities from acute fulminant hepatitis B are uncommon and occur in less than 1% of the patients who are so ill as to require hospitalization for hepatitis B infections.[51] Five percent to 10% of patients have a serum sickness–like illness related to vasculitis caused by circulating immune complexes of HBsAg/anti-HBsAg.[52] More commonly, the clinical disease is mild. Many patients with HBV infections do not become icteric.

**FIGURE 3-6** Typical clinical and serum findings of a patient with self-limited HBV infection. Hepatitis B virus antigens are present in serum early in the course of the infection. The antigens disappear as antibodies to HBV are produced.

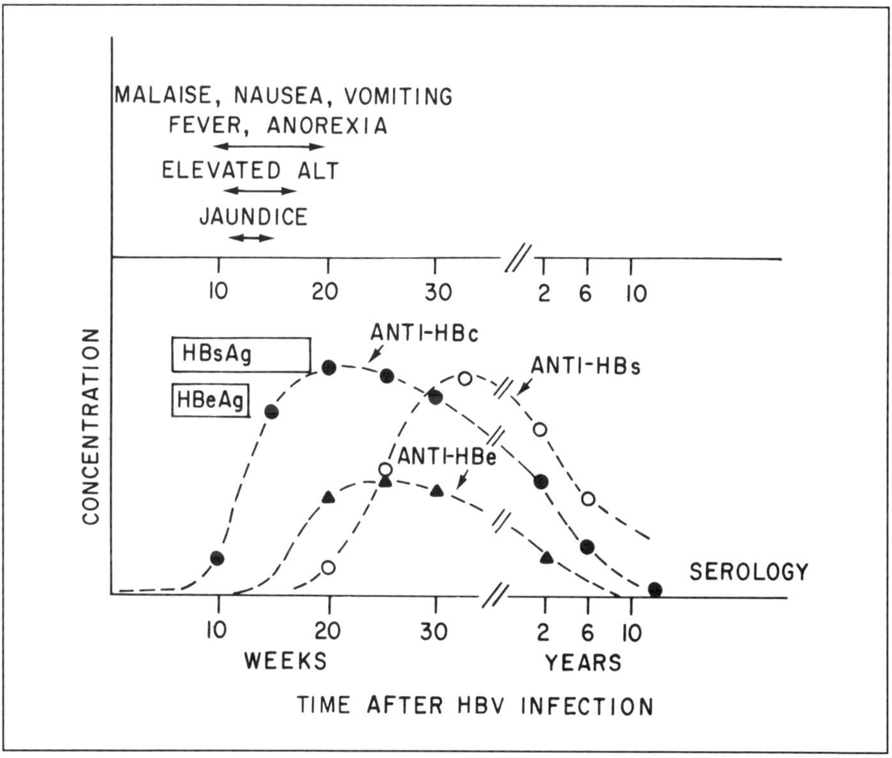


Antiviral antibodies are made in patients with self-limited disease. The first to appear is an antibody against core antigen, anti-HBc IgM, which usually can be detected 3 to 5 weeks after the appearance of HBsAg in the blood and before the onset of clinically apparent hepatitis.[20] Anti-HBC IgG is made several weeks later, after symptoms have occurred. In patients with self-limited disease, anti-HBC levels persist for weeks but fall to undetectable levels after the initial exposure. Antibody to HBsAg usually appears after antigenemia, during the convalescent period.[20] However, the antibody may be formed early, during antigenemia, with formation of antigen-antibody immune complexes. These immune complexes are found in patients with some of the extrahepatic manifestations of hepatitis B infection: rash, arthritis, and vasculitis.[52] The anti-HBsAg persists for years and is protective against reinfection.

**FIGURE 3-7** | Typical clinical and serum findings in chronic HBsAg carriers. Antigenemia persists; antibodies to HBs and HBe are not formed.

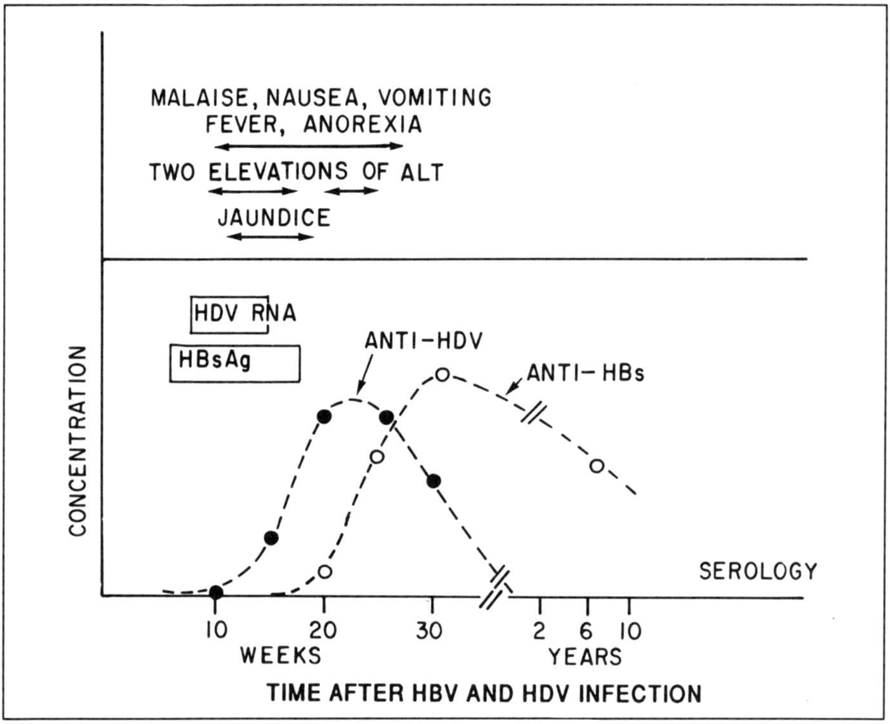


***Persistent Infections***

Some individuals infected with HBV do not produce antibody to HBsAg and do not clear HBsAg from serum. These patients have a prolonged (usually greater than 20 weeks) antigenemia and are termed chronic HBsAg carriers[20] (Figure 3-7). Persistent infection with HBV occurs in 10% of patients hospitalized with HBV. Individuals who are chronic carriers may be in good health and without persistent elevations of serum glutamic-oxaloacetic transaminase (SGOT) and serum glutamic pyruvate transaminase (SGPT). Histologically, the livers in the carriers are essentially normal aside from the presence of ground-glass hepatocytes that are associated with HBsAg.[53] Some chronic carriers have elevations in serum transaminase and histologically show chronic persistent hepatitis that is often benign and resolves in time. Others with elevated serum enzymes, about 5% of those infected, have chronic active hepatitis. These individuals may have jaundice with high transaminase levels.

The prognosis is variable. Some progress to cirrhosis; others have chronic infection, but the HBsAg is negative. Blood donors from this group of infected individuals, HBsAg negative, may transmit HBV infections by blood transfusions.[54,55]

**Typical Disease in the Transfused Individual**

The rates of posttransfusion hepatitis caused by HBV have been declining. In 1943, 18% of transfused patients had jaundice following a blood transfusion.[41] The mortality rate of patients with posttransfusion hepatitis was 19%. In 1962, Allen presented a similar 21% rate of posttransfusion hepatitis and 23% rate of mortality in patients older than 40 years of age.[56] When the Australia antigen was identified as a marker for hepatitis B, 75% of the recipients of Australia antigen–positive donor blood showed infection with HBV by the development of hepatitis or the appearance of anti-HBV antibodies.[57] The mortality rate was 3%. The elimination of units with Australia antigen and commercial blood donors brought down the rates of posttransfusion hepatitis from 18% to 3.3%.[44] Hepatitis B has not been prevented by these measures, and of the patients who still develop hepatitis, 39% develop hepatitis B.

Posttransfusion hepatitis B is usually icteric.[44] This compares to the low rate, 4%, of community-acquired hepatitis B that causes jaundice. More patients who acquire hepatitis B by transfusion have symptomatic infection with anorexia, fever, vomiting, and joint pain than those with community-acquired infection.[58] The mortality rate from posttransfusion hepatitis B is also greater than the disease acquired in the community. Posttransfusion mortality rates in patients with symptomatic hepatitis were high before the identification and exclusion of the Australia antigen, ranging from 12% to 23%.[41,59] Hepatitis B mortality in 1987 was 5% higher than the fatality rate in community-acquired disease, which is much less than 0.1%.[51,58]

Those who acquire hepatitis B by transfusion are also at risk for developing the carrier state with chronic HBsAg production. The risk of the development of the carrier state is greater in those with posttransfusion HBV infections. When HBV infection is acquired by a nontransfusion route, fewer than 10% of those infected become chronic HBV carriers. When HBV is transmitted by transfusion, the risk of the development of chronic HBV infection increases to 20%.

In summary, hepatitis B remains a significant cause of posttransfusion hepatitis, but the incidence has been reduced by screening techniques. The hepatitis caused by HBV is more symptomatic and has a higher mortality rate than HBV acquired by other routes. The risk that the HBV infection will become chronic is greater with posttransfusion HBV infection than the infection acquired by other routes.

### Steps Taken to Minimize the Risks

Donor selection to reduce the risk of hepatitis B infection begins with the history. Individuals with a history of hepatitis are excluded, as are those with a history of HBsAg. Since hepatitis B virus infections may occur in a similar population of individuals with HIV, the exclusion of those with high-risk behaviors (intravenous drug users, homosexual men, and prostitutes) will likely reduce transmission of hepatitis B as well as AIDS. Other screening questions about blood or body fluid exposure and accidental needle-stick injuries are also employed.[60]

Physical examination of the donors may eliminate those with evidence of needle tracts or sclerotic veins, which are suggestive of intravenous drug abuse. Tattoos may also be identified, and these should be more than 6 months old or the donor must be deferred. In the laboratory, all blood is tested for HBsAg, and positive units are not used for transfusion.[60]

### Infectivity of Blood Products

Hepatitis B is highly infectious. Inoculation by accidental needle-stick injury is well documented.[61] Hepatitis B has been identified in patients who have received blood, serum, or pooled plasma.[5,41,59]

## Delta Hepatitis

In 1977, a new antigen in hepatic nuclei was detected in patients with liver disease who were also chronically infected with HBV. An antibody to the antigen was found in the serum of these carriers of HBV.[62] A hepatitis virus, termed hepatitis D virus (HDV) or delta hepatitis, was responsible for the antigen (delta antigen) and caused the formation of anti-delta antigen. The virus was discovered to be a small RNA virus that acted as a parasite for HBV. Delta viral replication requires HBV enzymes. The HDV virion is formed by the encapsulation or HDV RNA in HBV and host-surface membranes.[63]

Because of its dependence on HBV, HDV infections occur in populations with HBV, and delta virus is transmitted by similar mechanisms.[64] Epidemiologic studies found a high prevalence of the virus in intravenous drug addicts and hemophiliacs treated with coagulation factors prepared by pooling plasma from many donors. Hepatitis D virus has also been found in the developing world where HBV is endemic.[65]

The risk of posttransfusion infection is low, because blood products are screened for HBsAg. Hemophiliacs treated with local plasma pools or single-donor plasma have a decreased risk of HDV infection compared to those hemophiliacs treated with commercially available pooled plasma.[66]

## Microbiology

The virion of HDV is a 36-nm spherical particle, which is coated by surface antigen of HBV (HBsAg). The core of the virion contains HDV RNA. The RNA is 5 x $10^5$ in molecular weight and is a single-stranded circle. It appears to be a negative RNA strand, because it cannot be directly translated in vitro and is unable to bind to ribosomes.[63] Two HDV proteins with delta antigenicity are identifiable in the core.

## Typical Disease in the Nontransfused Individual

Infection with HDV occurs in 1 of 2 clinical settings. An individual may be simultaneously infected with HBV and HDV and develop acute infectious HBV and HDV hepatitis. The second possibility is that a chronic carrier of HBV will become newly infected with HDV.

Acute hepatitis from HBV and HDV causes an illness similar clinically to HBV alone (Figure 3-8). After an incubation period characteristic of

**FIGURE 3-8** Typical clinical and serum findings in a patient with HBV and HDC coinfection.

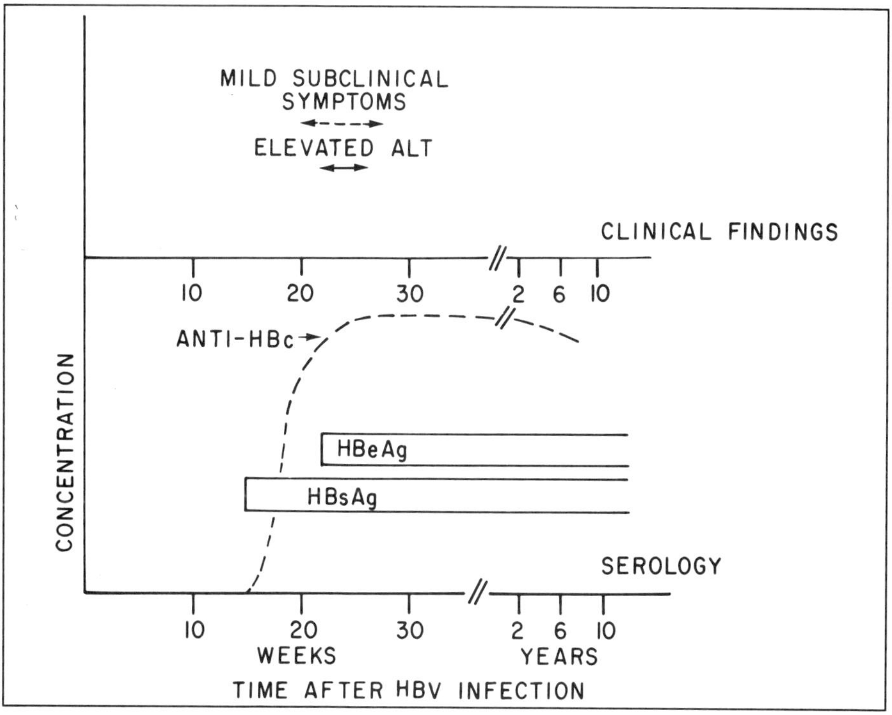

**FIGURE 3-9** | Typical clinical and serum findings in a chronic carrier of HBsAg who is subsequently superinfected with HDV.

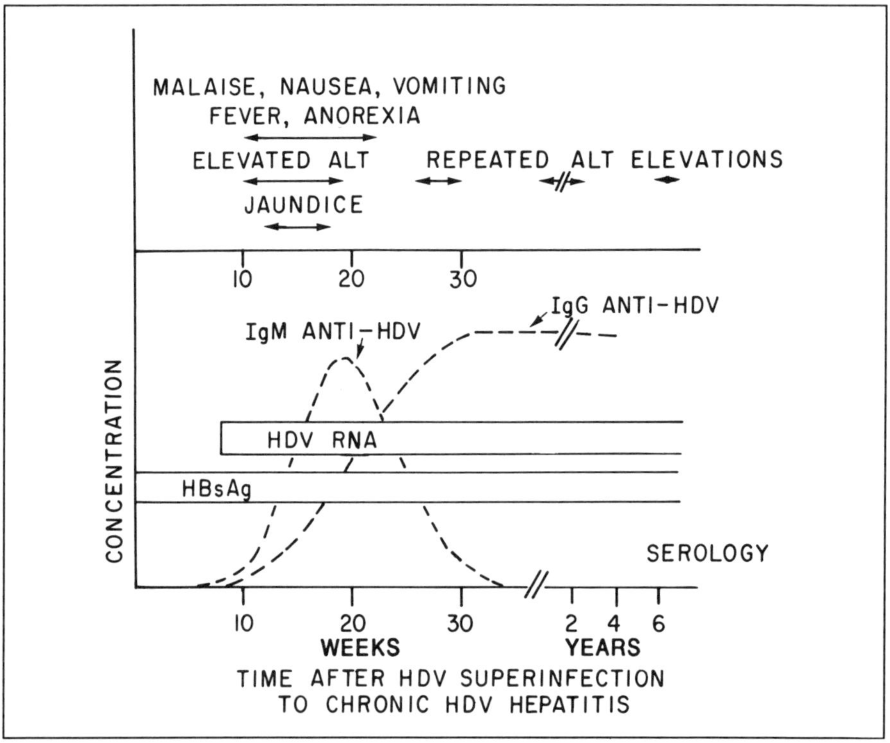


HBV, HBV is produced. Later, patients with HDV infection become symptomatic, have jaundice and abnormal hepatic enzymes, and develop an acute hepatitis that is clinically indistinguishable from that caused by other viruses.[63] Some patients have a biphasic increase in serum enzymes, with a second peak occurring 2 to 5 weeks after the first. Most patients recover uneventfully, and 4% become chronic carriers of HBV. Some of the cases of coinfection with HBV and HDV end in fulminant hepatitis and death. Mortality figures range from 0% to 17%,[63] and the rate of fulminant hepatitis and death is higher than HBV infection alone.

**Typical Disease in the Transfused Individual**

Previously transfused individuals who are chronic HBsAg carriers may become superinfected with HDV. The HDV is acquired in a similar manner as HBV. After an incubation period of 2 to 8 weeks, most (50%–70%) patients develop acute hepatitis. The severity of the hepatitis in HDV superinfection is greater than that of acute HBV hepatitis (Figure 3-9). Fulminant hepatitis is common, and the mortality rate approaches 20%.[65]

After the acute phase of the illness has passed, some patients will develop anti-HBsAg, and both the HBV and HDV will be cleared without residual disease. More commonly, infection with both viruses persists. Patients develop chronic liver disease, with elevated serum enzyme levels. Liver biopsy will show chronic active hepatitis or hepatitis that has progressed to cirrhosis.

### Steps Taken to Minimize the Risks

In 1965, Blumberg and colleagues[8] described an antigen that was found to be the surface antigen of HBV (HBsAg). Gocke's prospective studies, reported in 1970, clearly show an association between the transfusion of blood with HBsAg and the development of posttransfusion hepatitis.[57] Assays were developed to screen donor blood for HBsAg, and blood has been routinely screened for HBsAg since the 1970s.[67,68]

Since HDV requires the simultaneous infection with HBV to replicate, and because HDV uses surface membrane from HBV to form its virion,[69] one would expect that HDV would uncommonly be a cause of posttransfusion hepatitis. However, just as blood that is negative for HBsAg may cause posttransfusion HBV hepatitis, a risk for posttransfusion HDV does exist.[66,70] It is believed unlikely that additional screening for HDV would prevent HDV posttransfusion hepatitis.[59] In hemophiliacs the risk of HDV hepatitis has been reduced by the use of single-source or local donors rather than pooled commercial products.[66]

### Infectivity of Blood Products

It is assumed that HDV is as infectious as HBV and is transmitted in blood and plasma.

## Non-A, Non-B Hepatitis and Hepatitis C

Posttransfusion hepatitis has been the most serious infectious complication of blood transfusion. Epidemiologic studies in the 1940s to 1960s found that the risk of infection was significantly increased when the blood came from paid donors.[59,71] Patients receiving multiple-donor, pooled products also had higher rates of posttransfusion hepatitis. In 1965, the Australia antigen was discovered in the sera of transfused patients with leukemia[8] and later was shown to have a significant association with the infectivity of donor blood.[71,72] The Australia antigen has been found to be hepatitis B surface antigen

(HBsAg). The elimination of commercial blood donors and the universal donor screening for HBsAg have greatly reduced the incidence of posttransfusion hepatitis.[44,73,74]

However, these exclusion techniques have failed to eliminate posttransfusion hepatitis completely.[75,76] The hepatitis A virus was identified in the early 1970s,[12] and the discovery led to the development of methods for the diagnosis of HAV or "infectious hepatitis" infections.[34] Hepatitis A virus is an extremely rare cause of posttransfusion hepatitis.

Thus, the serologic and epidemiologic identification of hepatitis A and B failed to account for all of the known features of infectious hepatitis. Some patients were observed to have multiple attacks of acute hepatitis.[77] Other patients exhibited an incubation period for hepatitis intermediate to that of hepatitis A virus or hepatitis B virus.[78] Patients with HBsAg were observed to develop additional posttransfusion hepatitis, indicating that another non–hepatitis B virus was involved in transfusion hepatitis.[45,75]

The disease of non-A, non-B (NANB) posttransfusion hepatitis has been recognized. Three groups of blood donors were identified as having an increased risk of transmitting NANB hepatitis: paid donors, donors with an elevated serum alanine aminotransferase level (ALT), and donors with antibody to hepatitis B core antigen (anti-HBc).[79] The exclusion of paid donors and the use of these "surrogate tests" for identifying and excluding possible NANB infectious blood products have reduced the incidence of posttransfusion NANB hepatitis.[80,81]

In 1989, a report that the genome of a NANB hepatitis agent had been cloned and designated hepatitis C virus (HCV) was published by Choo and colleagues working at Chiron Corporation.[82] An accompanying report by the same group described an assay for antibodies to a virus causing NANB hepatitis.[83] When this assay was used to investigate serum of patients with posttransfusion NANB hepatitis, 70% to 90% of patients had the anti-HCV antibody.[83,84] Further, studies investigating the donors of patients who developed posttransfusion hepatitis also showed that 73% of the donors had anti-HCV antibody.[85-87] In addition, scientists at Chiron have developed a technique for HCV RNA testing using cDNA polymerase reaction.[100] The discovery of these 2 techniques promises to clarify the role that hepatitis C virus plays in NANB hepatitis.

## Microbiology

Before the identification of HCV, infectious NANB hepatitis had been studied in animal models. Posttransfusion hepatitis could be transmitted to chimpanzees by infected human blood products. By filtration and chemical studies, the infectious virus was found to be small, 30 to 60 nm in diameter, with a lipid envelope.[89] These physical properties suggested that the virus belonged to the viral family flavivirus. The nucleotide sequence of the HCV cDNA showed similarities to the flavivirus, but continued research will be required to classify HCV and define further its microbiology.[90]

### Typical Disease in the Nontransfused Individual

Non-A, non-B hepatitis, or HCV hepatitis, has been a serious infectious complication of transfusion of blood or blood products. The disease has also been recognized in patients without a history of parenteral exposure.[91,92] The criteria for the clinical diagnosis of NANB acute hepatitis are similar to those of HAV or HBV hepatitis. These include the clinical symptoms of hepatitis: malaise, anorexia, nausea, and vomiting (Figure 3-10). The serum ALT is elevated greater than 2.5 times the upper limit of normal. Other causes of liver injury, such as drugs, toxins, alcohol, heart failure, or malignancy, have been excluded. Serologic studies in a patient with acute NANB hepatitis are negative for the IgM antibodies to HAV and HBV.[91]

Many (39%) of the patients with nontransfusion NANB hepatitis give a history of intravenous drug use.[91] Another 5% had contact with an infected individual and had a history of multiple heterosexual partners. In 48% of patients, no specific source could be identified.

When the patients who had acute NANB hepatitis were tested for antibodies to HCV, 26% were positive.[91] In patients with NANB hepatitis that became chronic, 70% or more had antibodies to HCV. These data support the hypothesis that many cases of community-acquired NANB hepatitis were caused by HCV. Community-acquired NANB hepatitis often progresses to cirrhosis. A few patients with community-acquired HCV infections may recover completely, but more have stable persistent hepatitis or chronic active hepatitis with or without cirrhosis.[91,92] Of those with cryptogenic cirrhosis, approximately 70% have antibodies to HCV.

### Typical Disease in the Transfused Individual

Non-A, non-B hepatitis has been defined as the acute or chronic viral hepatitis in which serologic evidence of HAV or HBV exposure is negative, and no other cause of liver injury is apparent.[93] The disease is a form of serum hepatitis that has been spread by the parenteral route.[94] It has been a cause of posttransfusion hepatitis and is frequently seen in patients undergoing dialysis, hemophiliacs, medical care workers, and drug addicts.

Clinically acute NANB hepatitis is similar to acute hepatitis B. The mean incubation time is 50 days, ranging from 20 to 90 days. It is usually anicteric; only 25% of patients become jaundiced.[94] The death rate from acute NANB hepatitis is less than 1%. Antibody to

**FIGURE 3-10** Typical clinical and serum findings in a patient with hepatitis due to HCV. This virus causes repeated episodes of liver injury as measured by ALT. Hepatitis C virus often causes hepatic cirrhosis.

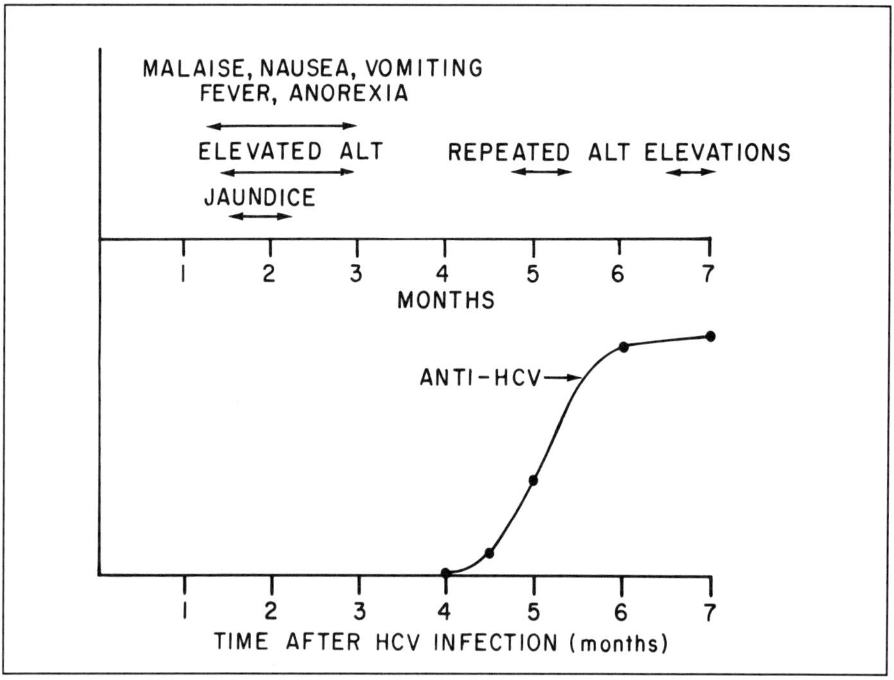


hepatitis C virus has been detected in 20% of cases of acute posttransfusion hepatitis.[84]

The clinical significance of NANB hepatitis is not the acute infection it causes, but rather the insidious and protracted chronic disease it becomes.[93] In prospective studies, 50% to 70% of patients with NANB hepatitis have biochemical evidence of chronic hepatitis, and 20% to 25% develop end-stage liver disease and hepatic cirrhosis. Because of the clinically unapparent or only mild acute hepatitis, transfusion-associated NANB hepatitis is often first diagnosed by symptoms of chronic liver disease. Chronic NANB hepatitis is 1 of the major causes of cirrhosis in the United States and is a frequent indication for liver transplantation.

One symptom of chronic active hepatitis is fatigue that has a slow onset, accompanied by anorexia, nausea, and vomiting. Fluctuating jaundice may be present. In some patients the complications of cirrhosis, such as ascites, bleeding esophageal varices, coagulopathy, or encephalopathy, cause the patient to seek medical care. The extrahepatic symptoms of urticaria, purpura, arthritis, or arthralgia are rarely seen.[93]

One laboratory feature in chronic NANB hepatitis is an increase in the serum levels of ALT and aspartate aminotransferase (AST). Enzyme levels remain elevated for a year or more.[95] The serum alkaline phosphate and γ-glutamyl transpeptidase values are elevated. Other abnormalities seen with cirrhosis and liver failure ensue, including thrombocytopenia, pancytopenia, and coagulopathy.

The histologic features of chronic NANB hepatitis are chronic active hepatitis in 60% of patients and chronic persistent hepatitis in 20%.[79] Long-term follow-up shows that 20% to 25% of patients with NANB hepatitis progress to hepatic cirrhosis.[95]

### Infectivity of Blood Products

Non-A, non-B hepatitis has been transmitted by many blood products. Transfusions of blood, packed RBCs, plasma, serum, cryoprecipitate, factor VIII concentrates, factor IX complex, and platelets have been followed by episodes of non-A, non-B hepatitis.[38]

### Steps Taken to Minimize the Risks

Surrogate markers for non-A, non-B hepatitis have been used to screen donor blood. The alarming aminotransferase levels correlate with the infectivity of donated blood products, as does the appearance of antibody to hepatis B core antigen.[96-99]

## CYTOMEGALOVIRUS

In the 1950s, a syndrome of anemia, leukocytosis with atypical lymphocytes, and fever began to be recognized in patients who had been transfused.[100] The disease differed from typical infectious mononucleosis by being heterophil negative. The syndrome, which occurred in patients following cardiac surgery, was termed a late-onset postperfusion mononucleosis. In 1966, a report described an increase in cytomegalovirus (CMV) antibodies in patients who had a heterophil-negative mononucleosis following blood transfusion.[101] A connection had been made between blood transfusion and the development of CMV mononucleosis. A mild posttransfusion CMV disease occurred in individuals in good health. A more serious concern was the development of CMV infections in the immunocompromised patient: the newborn, those with congenital immunodeficiency, or patients with acquired immunodeficiency due to AIDS, chemotherapy, or immunosuppression for organ transplantation. Studies have attempted to reduce the risk of posttransfusion CMV infection.[102]

## Microbiology

Cytomegalovirus is a member of the herpesvirus group.[103] The virion of CMV is the largest in the family, with a diameter of approximately 200 nm. The outer covering of CMV is a trilaminar lipid membrane envelope derived from the host cell membrane. There are 25 to 30 viral-encoded proteins and glycoproteins contained in the envelope. The envelope encloses the viral capsid, a 110-nm icosahedral structure formed by 162 viral capsomers. The CMV core contains the genome: linear double-stranded DNA. Cytomegalovirus has the largest genome of the herpesviruses.

Cytomegalovirus enters a cell following attachment to receptors by glycoproteins on the viral envelope. The viral capsid transverses the cell membrane and cytoplasm, and viral DNA is released into the nucleus. The alpha genes of viral DNA are transcribed and translated in the cytoplasm. The expression of the DNA to form these proteins is required for further DNA transcription.[103] At a later time, structural proteins are produced, and the viral DNA is replicated. Formed capsids with DNA assemble at the host cellular membrane, which has been modified by insertion viral proteins. The capsids are enveloped and released into the extracellular space.

The time for the synthesis of CMV is long compared to other herpesviruses. Maximal viral DNA production takes 72 to 96 hours. Cells productively infected with herpesvirus, that is, cells releasing virus, do not survive. The herpesvirus may, instead of reproducing, remain latent in the host cell only to be reactivated at a later time.

## Typical Disease in the Nontransfused Individual

Cytomegalovirus causes disease in several clinical settings. Cytomegalovirus is the most common agent of prenatal infection; the virus may infect a fetus during gestation and cause disease before birth.[104,105] Congenital CMV is recognized in 3000 to 4000 newborns per year in the United States. Another 4500 to 6000 children have handicaps secondary to neurologic injury caused by CMV infection in utero.[106]

A fetus may be delivered hydropic and stillborn from congenital CMV disease.[107] Other features of symptomatic congenital infection that may be diagnosed at birth include microcephalus or hydrocephalus, low birth weight, hepatomegaly with hepatitis and jaundice, splenomegaly with anemia and thrombocytopenia, and pneumonia. Additional studies may detect encephalitis, cerebral calcifications, and neurologic abnormalities.[108] Only 1 of 20 CMV-infected newborns shows serious symptoms at birth.[105] The asymptomatic CMV-infected neonate may have residual neurologic damage recognized later in childhood by deafness, mental retardation, paralysis, or convulsions.

The diagnosis of congenital CMV requires detection of the virus. A congenitally infected newborn will excrete virus at birth and for 3 to 4 weeks thereafter. An infant with a perinatal infection will not immediately shed virus; the virus cannot be cultured until after 3 to 4 weeks of life. The culture of virus from a neonate within the first 2 weeks after delivery allows the diagnosis of congenital CMV infection to be made.[109] Virus may be isolated from saliva or urine in the neonate. Viral antigens may be detected, or CMV infection may be diagnosed by identification of viral DNA in urine by a polymerase chain reaction.[109]

Cytomegalovirus infection of the fetus, neonate, or child may not cause disease.[104] In some children, acquired viral infection is associated with liver disease and splenomegaly. In these children, their chronic CMV infection causes hepatitis with an elevation of liver enzymes.[110]

Many adults in America and Western Europe were not infected with CMV as children.[111] CMV infection in adults causes a syndrome similar to Epstein-Barr virus.[112,113] The CMV infection in adults is characterized by fever, elevations in hepatic serum enzymes, and the appearance of atypical lymphocytes in the peripheral circulation. Cytomegalovirus mononucleosis differs from typical mononucleosis by being negative for the heterophil antibody.[113] Antibody to CMV, both IgG and IgM, rises in the first 2 weeks following the onset of symptoms, and anti-CMV IgG persists for years.[114,115]

Cytomegalovirus also causes disease in individuals whose normal immune status is impaired, including patients who have AIDS, transplanted organs, leukemia, leukopenia, and so on.[116] Commonly, cytomegalovirus mononucleosis is seen in these immunocompromised individuals. Patients have fever, hepatic enzyme elevation, and peripheral lymphocytosis.[114,115]

The next most commonly diagnosed disease in the immunosuppressed person is cytomegalovirus pneumonitis.[116] The most common symptoms are fever, dyspnea, and nonproductive cough. The chest radiographs show an interstitial infiltrate. Histologically the lung has edema, fibrosis, alveolar exudate, and cells infected with CMV. Cytomegalovirus hepatitis is also frequently seen in the organ transplant patient. Patients have hepatomegaly, jaundice, and abnormal liver function tests.[117] This disease may improve without specific treatment. Cytomegalovirus gastroenteritis is especially severe in patients with AIDS with colitis, diarrhea, esophagitis, dysphagia, anal disease, pain, and gastrointestinal bleeding. Cytomegalovirus chorioretinitis may impair normal vision.

## Typical Disease in the Transfused Individual

Blood recipients differ in their risk for CMV disease depending on their underlying immune status. Immunocompetent seropositive patients who receive blood products are asymptomatic for CMV disease but may show an increase in their titer of anti-CMV antibody.[102] Some seronegative immunocompetent individuals who received a large amount of fresh blood, as was seen with open heart transplant patients in the early days of bypass surgery, developed a posttransfusion CMV mononucleosis. The incidence of CMV infection in this patient population before 1972 was 16% to 67%. These patients with CMV mononucleosis recovered without sequelae. Most patients with transfusion-related CMV disease were asymptomatic.

Immunocompromised patients who receive blood are at greater risk for symptomatic disease. Newborn infants, especially those of low birth weight, are at risk for posttransfusion CMV disease. A syndrome similar to CMV mononucleosis has been described in these preterm infants.[118] The infants had gray pallor, respiratory deterioration, hepatosplenomegaly, and atypical lymphocytosis. The mortality was 21% of the CMV-infected premature infants. Other studies have shown that the infection rates for CMV in blood-transfused low–birth weight newborns ranged from a high of 32% to a low of 2%, and most showed an infectious rate of less than 10%.[118]

Patients who receive organ transplantation of kidneys, heart, bone marrow, or liver are immunosuppressed and at risk for CMV infections. Blood products may cause infection in serologically negative graft recipients. Symptomatic disease varies from CMV mononucleosis to disseminated fatal infections.

Patients with AIDS are also at risk for transfusion-related CMV disease. Many adults with AIDS are seropositive and protected from infection. Children with AIDS, those with congenital infection, or hemophiliacs may be seronegative and at risk.

### Steps Taken to Minimize the Risks

The immunocompetent blood recipient is usually not at risk for symptomatic CMV infection. Cytomegalovirus antibody is not routinely assayed. In epidemiologic surveys, rates of seropositivity of donors range from 17% to 89%. Older donors and women are more likely to have prior viral exposure.

One proven method to decrease the risk of posttransfusion CMV infection is to use only seronegative blood in patients at risk. Another method is to wash the cells, such as is done for frozen deglycerolized RBCs. Older blood is no safer than fresh blood.[102]

### Infectivity of Blood Products

Pooled granulocytes have a greater risk of CMV infection than other products. Platelet preparations also contain granulocytes. Whole blood and packed RBCs have more risk than washed frozen RBCs. Techniques being studied for use are centrifugation and filtering of blood units.[102,121,122] Fresh frozen plasma has not been found to transmit CMV infection.[123]

## Epstein-Barr Virus

Epstein-Barr virus (EBV) was discovered in 1964 during the electron microscopic studies of Burkitt's lymphoma, a tumor of African children.[124] The virus is responsible for infectious mononucleosis in adults and children.[125] Epstein-Barr virus was recognized in the late 1960s as a cause of transfusion-associated illness. Postperfusion syndrome, a disease similar to mononucleosis, was diagnosed in patients who had blood transfusions during open heart surgery.[126] Most of these cardiac patients were found to have CMV infections, but EBV has caused the postperfusion syndrome in a small number of patients.[126] Most adults are seropositive with antibodies against EBV.[127] Since infectious mononucleosis is a benign, self-limited disease, without sequelae, and because most adults are immune to EBV, it is not considered a serious posttransfusion disease.[128]

## Microbiology

Epstein-Barr virus is a DNA virus of the herpesvirus family.[129] It has a structure similar to other herpesviruses with a DNA protein core that has the EBV nuclear antigen (EBNA) and a nucleocapsid with the viral capsid antigen (VCA). These structures are enveloped by a tegmentum and outer membrane. The virus replicates in epithelial cells of the oropharynx and B lymphocytes.[129]

The virus enters cells via surface receptors. In lymphocytes the receptor is thought to be a complement receptor, termed CD21.[126] After the virus enters the cell, its DNA is transported to the host cell nucleus. The virus may remain latent in the cell or may undergo replication. In an infected individual, viral shedding may continue for months.[129]

## Serology

A feature of infection by EBV is the host production of heterophil antibodies; these are antibodies that agglutinate sheep erythrocytes. Fewer than 10% of cases of infectious mononucleosis are negative for the heterophil antibody. Specific EBV antigens may also be detected.[130] Serum IgM antibody to EBV capsid antigen is transiently produced for 1 to 2 months following the primary EBV infection. IgG to VCA is produced, and moderately high titers of the antibodies persist for years. Antibodies against other viral proteins are also formed.[127]

## Typical Disease in the Nontransfused Individual

Infectious mononucleosis is the disease caused by EBV. Its incubation period is 30 to 50 days.[125,131] A prodromal period occurs with mild symptoms of headache, malaise, and fatigue, followed by fever, sore throat, and tender lymphadenopathy. About half of the patients with acute infectious mononucleosis have splenomegaly, and splenic rupture is a rare fatal complication of the disease.[131]

The patients have an increased number of circulating lymphocytes, with the appearance of atypical lymphocytes. Heterophil antibodies develop in the first week of the disease. Other antibodies to EBV antigens are detected, including IgM to EBV-VCA, IgG to EBV-VCA, and other antibodies.[127] Infectious mononucleosis usually lasts 2 to 3 weeks, and patients recover uneventfully.[129]

Seroconversion in children, especially those younger than 2 years of age, is generally not accompanied by symptomatic disease.[125] Occasionally, the children may have nonspecific findings of upper respiratory tract infection with cough, lymphadenopathy, pharyngitis, vomiting, or diarrhea. In children, like adults, recovery is usually uneventful.

### Typical Disease in the Transfused Individual

Healthy blood donors are found to shed EBV into their oral secretions, and viral-infected B lymphocytes have been identified in their peripheral blood.[130] As most donors were infected with EBV in childhood, 94% to 99% have IgG antibodies to EBV.[130,132] Because of this, patients may acquire EBV infections following blood transfusion.

A mononucleosislike illness may occur after the infusion of blood or blood products in patients who lack antibody to EBV.[132] The incubation period reported has varied from 17 days in a patient with leukemia receiving platelet-rich plasma to 57 days in a young woman receiving fresh whole blood during a splenectomy. The average incubation period is 35 to 48 days.[131]

Some patients who seroconvert for EBV after transfusion are asymptomatic. Others show more typical signs and symptoms of infectious mononucleosis with fever, splenomegaly, lymphadenopathy, circulating atypical lymphocytes, and the formation of heterophil antibodies.[131] Transfusion-related EBV infection in the older patient causes fever and malaise, without the typical pharyngitis, cervical adenopathy, or splenomegaly seen in young adults with infectious mononucleosis.[133] Patients with EBV infection acquired by transfusion may have morbidity due to fever, malaise, and other symptoms, but no patient has been described to die of the infection.

### Steps Taken to Minimize the Risks

Prospective blood donors undergo a screening process in which questions are asked to determine if they have an acute EBV illness. Patients who are symptomatic for infectious mononucleosis would be deferred for their fever, malaise, and other features of the disease. It is difficult to eliminate EBV in donor units, because many asymptomatic blood donors have EBV in circulating lymphocytes. For this reason, and because of the mildness of posttransfusion EBV infection, further studies are not done to minimize the possibility of contracting the disease following transfusion.[133]

### Infectivity of Blood Products

Most reports of posttransfusion EBV infection have described the disease following the transmission of blood.[132,134] One report documented EBV infection following the transfusion of platelet-rich plasma.

## Human T-cell Lymphotropic Virus

Viruses have long been known to cause malignancies and leukemias in animals.[135] The first virus associated with human malignancies was the retrovirus, HTLV, which was isolated from a patient with a lymphoid T-cell malignancy. This virus is endemic in some parts of the world and has been associated with 2 diseases: adult T-cell leukemia/lymphoma (ATL), which is malignant, and a nonneoplastic neurologic disease, tropical spastic paraparesis (TSP), also called HTLV-I–associated myelopathy (HAM). Adult T-cell leukemia has not been reported to occur following a blood transfusion, but blood transfusions have been associated with the development of the HTLV-I–related myelopathy.[136] In addition, HTLV-I is in the family of HIV. For these reasons, the laboratory testing of blood donor samples to exclude HTLV-I carriers has been implemented.[137]

### Microbiology

HTLV-I is a single-stranded RNA virus. Its genome codes for viral coat proteins in the *gag* region, polymerase in the *pol* region, and surface envelope proteins in the *envl* region. The proteins encoded in the *gag* region are the precursor p55 and proteins p19 and p24. The *envl* region encodes the precursor glycoprotein gp 61/68 and the proteins gp 21 and gp 46.

The virus binds to helper/inducer lymphocyte via the CD4 receptor and is internalized. The virus undergoes transcription to form a resultant DNA provirus. The DNA is inserted into human DNA at sites on the genome that vary from patient to patient. Viral infection is associated with the proliferation of T cells.[138] The virus may remain latent in the infected cell. On activation, the proviral DNA is transcribed to make viral proteins and to form RNA for the daughter cells. The virus is assembled and buds off the lymphocyte cell membranes.[139]

### Typical Disease in the Nontransfused Individual

Infection with HTLV-I is not often associated with the development of disease. The virus is found in Africa, southern Japan, the Caribbean, and the southeastern United States. In healthy residents in Japan, the rate of seropositivity is about 15%.[140-142] In the Caribbean, the overall rate is 5%. The rates of seropositivity increase with age and are greater in women. In the United States, the rate in healthy blood donors is only 0.025%.

Two diseases have been associated with infection by HTLV-I. The first of these, a chronic, degenerative, neurologic disease,[142,143] has been termed tropical spastic paraparesis (TSP) and HTLV-I–associated myelopathy (HAM). The disease is a slowly progressive myelopathy that involves mainly the pyramidal tracts. The symptoms and signs include progressive leg weakness with spasticity as well as sensory disturbances, back pain, urinary incontinence, and impotence. HAM/TSP has a peak occurrence in patients who are 40 to 50 years of age but has occurred in all age groups. The disease is more frequently seen in women than in men. Histologically, chronic inflammatory cells are noted around vessels in the meninges, white and gray matter of the brain, involving the myelin sheaths. The inflammation is described as a chronic diffuse leukomyelitis. The disease has been treated with steroids, with some response. It is estimated that only 1 of 2000 or 3000 carriers of HTLV will develop HAM.[144]

The second disease associated with HTLV, and the one from which the virus was isolated, is adult T-cell leukemia/lymphoma.[138] In the asymptomatic or subclinical phase of the disease, the virus may be detected by the individual's seropositivity or by proviral incorporation in lymphocytes. There may be circulating abnormal lymphocytes.

As the disease progresses to a chronic or smoldering phase, cutaneous lesions appear as erythematous papules and nodules. The numbers of circulating abnormal lymphocytes may increase. The bone marrow involvement with abnormal cells is only slight. Serum studies show an increase in immunoglobulins. This stage may be maintained for long periods of time.

As the disease continues, patients may have more symptoms, including rash, cough, weakness, fevers, and malaise. Lymph nodes increase in size, and hepatosplenomegaly is noted. Abnormal lymphocytes continue to circulate and are found in the cerebrospinal fluid. The lungs often have leukemic infiltrates, and opportunistic infections are seen. Many patients have lytic lesions in the long bones and skull. Serum calcium levels are elevated.[138] Once this phase of the disease has been identified, the malignancy can be treated with chemotherapy. Remissions are brief, and survival is limited. This malignant process is estimated to occur in 1 in 1700 patients infected with the virus.[141,142,145] In endemic areas of Japan and the West Indies, 40% to 60% of newly diagnosed lymphomas are caused by HTLV-I.

### Typical Disease in the Transfused Individual

Adult T-cell leukemia has not been described as an infectious complication of transfusion. This may be because of a long period of viral latency, since HTLV-I has only been identified for the last 10 years. The HTLV-

I–associated malignancy may require longer than 10 years to develop. Transfused patients exposed to HTLV-I may in the future be found to have adult T-cell leukemia.

The neurologic disease tropical spastic paraparesis (TSP), also termed HTLV-I–associated myelopathy (HAM), has been transmitted by transfusion. Three of 16 Japanese patients described by Shibasaki and associates[143] had received blood transfusions 2 to 19 years before developing the disease. In the United States, Saxton and associates[136] described a man who had received multiple blood transfusions following a motor vehicle accident. A year later he had symptoms of HAM with seropositivity for HTLV-I and proviral DNA in his mononuclear cells. Seroconversion has occurred in 63% of those receiving whole blood, packed RBCs, and platelets.[146] The disease has not been spread by cell-free blood products or fresh frozen plasma, and it has not been reported in hemophiliacs treated with pooled products.[140]

### Steps Taken to Minimize the Risks

At present, blood is routinely tested for human T-cell lymphotropic virus by serologic means. An enzyme-linked immunosorbent assay (ELISA) of the donor's blood, when repeatedly positive, is an indication for permanent donor deferment. In the United States, the incidence of HTLV infection in healthy blood donors is 0.025% to 0.38%, as studied by ELISA.[145,147] In Hawaii, 0.2% of healthy blood donors were positive for HTLV, and all of these donors were Japanese.[137] In Japan, the donor incidence rate is 2%.[146]

### Infectivity of Blood Products

Infection with HTLV has only followed the transfusion of blood products with cells: blood, packed RBCs, and platelets. It has not been reported following the transfusion of plasma or hemophilic concentrates.[137]

## Human Immunodeficiency Virus

A new immunodeficiency disease began to be recognized in the early 1980s.[148,149] The disease occurred in young male homosexuals and intravenous drug abusers who had previously been well. The patients were contracting infections such as *Pneumocystis carinii* pneumonia, mucosal candidiasis, and multiple viral infections usually only seen in the clinical settings of T-cell deficiency or immunosuppressive therapy.[148,150] The patients were anergic (ie, they lacked a cutaneous response to common antigens and had an inversion in their plasma lymphocyte T helper-to-suppressor ratio). In normal individuals the ratio is 1.6, in the patients studied the ratio was as low as 0.01.[148] Some had Kaposi's sarcoma, which is unusual in young males.[151] The Centers for Disease Control (CDC) established criteria to define the acquired immunodeficiency syndrome (AIDS) and began to accept reports of the illness in the United States in 1983.[152]

The occurrence of the disease in homosexual males and intravenous drug users suggested parenteral routes of transmission similar to that of hepatitis B. Reports of AIDS occurring in patients with hemophilia further indicated an infection that could be spread in contaminated blood products.[153,154] Since the infectious agent was unknown, and although there was no absolute evidence that AIDS was transmitted by blood products, these reported cases raised the concern in blood centers, transfusion services, and public health agencies. There was a fear that the nation's blood supply was contaminated and that transfusions could spread AIDS.[155]

An attempt was made to reduce the risks of acquiring AIDS in blood products. Physicians were urged to balance their decisions to transfuse blood against its infectious risk. Autologous blood transfusions with the patient's previously donated blood or blood recovered at the patient's surgery were suggested as alternates to allogenic, banked blood for elective surgeries. It was recommended that the donor screening process be modified to include questions that would detect symptoms of AIDS and elicit a history of belonging to a group who has a high prevalence of the disease.[156] These changes in the donor screening process increased the number of deferments. In New York, the questions were found to increase donor deferment and to reduce the number of male donors. More donors indicated that their donated blood should not be used for patient transfusion but only for laboratory use.[157] On review, the blood donated for research rather than transfusion had an increased incidence of hepatitis B core antibody and a 20 to 100 times greater frequency of HIV antibody.[158]

In 1984, reports began to be published that viruses from the human T-cell lymphotropic retrovirus (HTLV) family were associated with AIDS.[159-161] Following the identification of a virus in patients with AIDS, methods were developed to detect seropositivity. In 1985, the Food and Drug Administration (FDA) issued a license for an enzyme-linked immunoassay (EIA) for the human T-cell lymphotropic virus type III (HTLV-III), and testing for HTLV-III was immediately begun by the American Red Cross and other blood centers.[162] Samples that were repeatedly positive by EIA were further tested by a Western blot (WB) analysis. Overall, 0.038% of the blood donors in the United States were positive by EIA and WB (EIA+/WB+). In communities with a higher prevalence of AIDS, the prevalence of EIA+/WB+ was higher: 0.11%. When donors who tested positive by EIA and WB were interviewed, 88% were in 1 of the following groups: homosexual or bisexual males, intravenous drug users and their sexual partners, recently transfused patients, and males with heterosexual activity with African prostitutes.[163,164]

## Microbiology

AIDS is caused by the retrovirus, human immunodeficiency virus (HIV-1), formerly called HTLV-III. This virus is an enveloped RNA.[160] The surface of the virion has the viral proteins gp120 and gp41 and components of the host cell membranes. In the viral core are the major core proteins, p7, p9, p17, and p24, and the viral enzymes, reverse transcriptase, endonuclease, and a protease.

The viral genome has been characterized. The *gag* region produces the proteins of the viral core. The *pol* region transcribes the viral region, and the *env* region codes the envelope glycoproteins. The remaining regions of the genome code for the regulatory proteins of viral replication. Areas on the gene serve as junctional points for the integration of the proviral DNA genome into host DNA.[165]

The virus enters host cells by 1 of 2 mechanisms. The first method is the binding of the surface glycoprotein gp120 to the host cell's surface protein CD4, a high-affinity receptor for the virus. The CD4 protein is present in highest density on helper T lymphocytes (T4) and is found on some other cells such as monocytes and macrophages. The second method is not so clearly defined. In cell culture, some cells without CD4 surface proteins can be infected, indicating an additional mechanism for viral entry into cells. However, the infection of the T4 lymphocyte results in the profound immunosuppression that characterizes the disease in AIDS.[164,165]

Once bound to the CD4 receptor, the viral core is internalized into the host cytoplasm. The genomic viral RNA is transcribed by the reverse transcriptase enzyme to form double-stranded proviral DNA. The DNA accumulates in the cytoplasm or passes into the nucleus where it becomes integrated into the host DNA. The virus may remain latent in the infected cell, with little production of viral RNA or protein. Once the HIV genome has been integrated into the host DNA, the host cell is infected for life. The HIV infection may be productive, and virions are produced by the host cell. The proviral DNA serves as template for both mRNA and genomic RNA. Translation of the mRNA occurs with protein synthesis. The proteins are processed, and the virus is assembled. Release occurs by budding of mature virions on the cell surface.[165,166]

Infection with HIV is associated with depletion of the circulating T cells that express the CD4 phenotype. In cell culture, production of the HIV virion by T cells is associated with cytopathic changes. Cells become multinucleated, show balloon degeneration, and eventually die. It is not known if these degenerative cytopathic events occur in the infected host, but the reduction of CD4 T cells regularly accompanies the symptoms of AIDS. During the productive infection, virus is found in the blood and cerebrospinal fluid at levels of 10 to 50 infectious particles per milliliter. Virus is also found in cells in seminal fluid and in vaginal and cervical fluids and has been isolated in breast milk. The virus may be passed from an infected mother to a fetus.[164,165]

## Identification and Serology

One method of diagnosing HIV infection is the direct isolation of the virus. For the assay, uninfected T lymphocytes are isolated and cocultured with peripheral blood lymphocytes from the patient at risk for HIV.[167] Identification of the retrovirus is made by the detection of characteristic reverse transcriptase in the supernatant of the cultured cells. Microscopic examination of the cultured cells may detect viral particles.[159] Viral cultures may diagnose HIV infection in those without serum titers of anti-HIV antibodies.[167,168] These methods are not routinely used to diagnose HIV infection because they require the prolonged culture of human T cells, which take 3 to 9 weeks to show signs of infection. The procedure is further handicapped because it lacks sensitivity; viruses cannot be consistently isolated from symptomatic patients with AIDS.

More commonly tests are used that identify viral antigens or detect antiviral antibodies. HIV viral antigen or genome may be detected in the peripheral blood of an individual before the individual seroconverts with the formation of anti-HIV IgM or IgG.[169,170] Viral DNA in host cells also may be detected. The small amount of viral genome in the infected host cells may be increased for in vitro analysis by enzymatic amplification of specific regions of the host and HIV genome.[171,172] The specific identification of HIV genome is made by utilizing a labeled probe for the portion of amplified region. The DNA is cleaved by a specific restriction endonuclease, and the characteristic fragments are identified after electrophoresis. This technique may identify HIV genome in as short a time as 3 or 4 days. In HIV seronegative individuals at risk for AIDS, HIV provirus may be present in the host cells for months to years before seroconversion.[169] Alternatively, early HIV infection may be diagnosed in individuals who have not produced antibodies by the identification of viral antigens, often the core protein p24 and the surface protein gp41.[172]

Following viral infection, anti-HIV IgM is found to be produced before the synthesis of anti-HIV IgG, and identification of antiviral IgM has been made in individuals seronegative for IgG. In those infected who have a complete battery of screening tests, viral antigen is produced, rising to a peak before the detection of antibody.[173] IgM is produced 1 to 2 weeks after the identification of viral antigen and is seen to increase as the viral antigen titer decreases. Within weeks after IgM is identified, seroconversion for anti-HIV IgG occurs.[173] The identification of anti-HIV IgM in an infant allows diagnosis of infection, in the presence of maternal transplacental serum IgG.[174]

The screening test most commonly used to detect antibody to HIV in serum is the enzyme-linked immunosorbent assay (ELISA).[175] The ELISA may be falsely positive due to cross-reacting antibodies, including anti-HLA antibodies in the serum of multiparous women or previously transfused patients.[176] Most laboratories testing for antibodies against HIV antigens will repeat the test of a positive serum sample by the ELISA method and then confirm the specificity of the antibody by a Western blot analysis to detect antibodies to the HIV antigens p24, gp41, and gp120/160.[175] The p24 antigen is the HIV *gag* protein, gp41 is a transmembrane envelope glycoprotein, and gp120/160 are *env* glycoproteins.

**Typical Disease in the Nontransfused Individual**

The acquired immunodeficiency syndrome was first recognized in the early 1980s in drug abusers and homosexuals who had contracted infectious diseases such as *Pneumocystis carinii* pneumonia or chronic herpes simplex ulcers. These patients had additional opportunistic infections with *Candida*, cytomegalovirus, and *Mycobacterium avium*.[149,152] These infections are unusual outside the settings of congenital immunodeficiency or immunosuppressive chemotherapy for malignant neoplastic diseases and organ transplantation. The infections had developed in individuals who were previously well, suggesting an acquired condition that had impaired normal T-cell function. In 1982, the Centers for Disease Control received reports that similar opportunistic infections were occurring in hemophiliacs receiving factor VIII concentrates.[152] These observations suggested an infectious etiology, which has been confirmed by the isolation of the HIV virus.

Many of the clinical features of AIDS are directly related to compromise of helper T4 lymphocyte function. The virus binds to the CD4 molecule on the surface, infects the nuclei, and has a cytopathic effect that reduces the numbers and functional abilities of the T4 lymphocytes. T4 lymphocytes have a critical role in the normal human immune response.[165] Activated T4 cells release lymphokines that have effects on other cells. T4 cells release interleukin-II (IL-2), which activates natural killer cells, cytotoxic T cells, monocytes, and macrophages. IL-2 activates B lymphocytes to promote their growth and differentiation to plasma cells. Other lymphokines normally released by activated T4 cells affect the growth of hematopoietic stem cells, mast cells, and fibroblasts.[165]

Individuals infected with HIV have decreased numbers of T4 lymphocytes and show abnormalities of T4 functions, such as decreased cellular proliferative responses to soluble antigens, impaired delayed hypersensitivity response, decreased helper function, and decreased humoral response to immunization.[177] Those individuals with HIV disease acquire opportunistic infections and other illnesses related to immunoincompetence. In addition, HIV infects cells other than T lymphocytes, with the additional consequences of neurologic and gastrointestinal dysfunction.[165]

Men, women, and children have acquired AIDS by mechanisms other than by transfusion of blood or blood products.[178] Most (70%) of the men who have community-acquired AIDS are homosexual or bisexual. Some are intravenous drug users or both homosexual and intravenous drug users. Infection acquired in men by heterosexual sex occurs infrequently in the United States. Most of the women with AIDS are intravenous drug abusers or heterosexual partners of those with or at risk for AIDS. Nearly all of the children with AIDS have acquired the disease through a parent.

**Manifestations of AIDS**

Infection with HIV results in a spectrum of clinical conditions, from the asymptomatic carrier to the patient dying of AIDS. The Centers for Disease Control has established criteria in diagnosing AIDS.[152,179] These criteria include the following: the acquisition of an opportunistic infection, such as candidiasis, *Mycobacterium avium, Pneumocystis carinii,* and others, in the setting of HIV infection; the acquisition of malignancies such as Kaposi's sarcoma or lymphoma; and the development of an encephalopathy or a wasting syndrome. Infected persons with persistent generalized lymphadenopathy are said to have AIDS-related complex (ARC), classified as a Group III infection. Group II infections include those individuals classified as infected but asymptomatic. Group I infections occur with the initial infection that often has a mononucleosislike illness. Similar classification criteria have been developed for children.[180]

***Initial Infection, Group I***

Diagnosis of HIV by ELISA or WB is not possible early in HIV infection, because individuals have not seroconverted with production of anti-HIV IgM and IgG. In high-risk individuals, an acute viral syndrome has been identified.[181] The patients exhibited symptoms such as fevers, rash, myalgia-arthralgias, and pharyngitis. These symptoms spontaneously resolved in 8 to 12 days. HIV antigen was detected in the acute phase of the illness, and convalescent sera drawn 6 to 30 days after the acute illness were positive for anti-HIV core and anti-HIV *env.* Class I infection may not be diagnosed, because the symptoms are nonspecific and initial serum testing may not be done. After the acute phase of the illness has passed, the individual may be reclassified as the disease progresses into Group II, III, and IV.

***Chronic Asymptomatic Infection, Group II***

Often individuals may be infected without clinical evidence of disease. A latent period between infection and illness may last for years.[177] Viral infection and antigenemia may precede seroconversion for years as well.[168-170]

Before symptoms or signs of disease develop, immune function can be tested in infected individuals. Early in the course of AIDS, the number of CD4+ cells and the CD4/CD8 (T-cell helper to T-cell suppressor) ratio are normal. B-cell function is normal. The CDC continues to classify these individuals as Group II A, asymptomatic infection.

The progression of the infection, however, is associated with an attrition of the numbers of T4 cells. This decline varies greatly from 1 individual to another.[164]

In time, abnormalities of the immune system are detected, including the decrease in the numbers of T4 cells, abnormalities in B-cell function, polyclonal B-cell activation, and hypergammaglobulinemia. Immune complexes and autoantibodies appear in the serum.[177] Functional assays of cellular immunity become abnormal; proliferative responses to pokeweed and other mitogens decrease. When abnormal immune function is detected, the individual is considered Group II B by CDC classifications. When symptoms develop, the infection is classified as Group III or IV.

### *Symptoms That Fail to Classify as Full-Blown AIDS, Group III*

Patients have fever, weight loss, diarrhea, fatigue, and night sweats. Persistent generalized lymphadenopathy may be found in addition to serologic evidence of infection and immunologic abnormalities. This period of the infection has been termed the AIDS-related complex (ARC). Many conditions proceed to AIDS, although some patients have died of the wasting syndrome without having signs or symptoms required to diagnose AIDS.[177]

### *AIDS, Group IV*

As the disease progresses, patients acquire opportunistic infections and develop prolonged constitutional symptoms of fever, weight loss, and neurologic dysfunction. HIV infection involves many organ systems, but most prominent are diseases of the lungs and the brain. Differences in AIDS in adults and children exist, and the kinds of diseases encountered will be discussed separately.

Pulmonary abnormalities are a major source of morbidity and mortality in AIDS. More than half of patients with AIDS have significant pulmonary disease.[182,183] Both community-acquired and opportunistic pulmonary infections are common in patients with AIDS. In decreasing order of frequency, *Pneumocystis carinii* pneumonia, cytomegalovirus pneumonia, *Mycobacterium avium-intracellulare*, and bacterial infections with *Haemophilus influenzae* and *Streptococcus pneumoniae* are seen. *Pneumocystis carinii* pneumonia is the major opportunistic infection, both as the primary infection to make the diagnosis of AIDS in 64% of patients and occurring at least once in 80% of patients with AIDS.[182] Recurrent *Pneumocystis* pneumonia is common, as are concurrent multiple pulmonary infections. Many patients with AIDS die of respiratory failure caused by these infections, despite treatment with antibiotics and respiratory support with mechanical ventilation.

Other noninfectious pulmonary complications are seen in patients with AIDS. Malignancies are common in patients infected with HIV, and these involve the lung. Kaposi's sarcoma is the most common malignancy seen, occurring in up to 40% of homosexual men with the disease.[183] About one half of those with Kaposi's sarcoma have pulmonary involvement. Median survival after the development of the sarcoma is variably reported, ranging from 2 to 10 months,[182] but some patients survive as long as several years.

In addition to the pulmonary involvement of Kaposi's sarcoma, other malignancies seen in patients with AIDS cause pulmonary disease. Malignancies such as non-Hodgkin's lymphoma, Hodgkin's lymphoma, and hematologic malignancies occur in lungs and involve the thoracic viscera.[184]

The pulmonary condition, lymphoid interstitial pneumonitis, is a chronic inflammatory and infiltrative disease. The lymphocytes do not infiltrate the lungs as a consequence of infection or malignancy.[182] Patients have progressive dyspnea with nodular infiltrates on the chest radiograph. In the lung, a pleomorphic cell population of lymphocytes, plasma cells, and immunoblasts infiltrates the pulmonary parenchyma. In some patients with AIDS, the disease has responded to steroids, with improvement of respiratory function. In others, steroid treatment has been associated with worsening lung disease due to secondary infection with organisms such as *Haemophilus influenzae, Staphylococcus aureus,* and *Streptococcus pneumoniae.*

After the pulmonary diseases, diseases of the nervous system cause major morbidity and mortality in patients with AIDS. In contrast to the pulmonary diseases, in which the impact of AIDS is secondary to immunosuppression, the neurologic disease is related directly to the viral infection of the brain.[185,186] This viral infection is similar to the viral infections in animal models of neurodegenerative disease.

In the early stage of the HIV infection, the virus enters the brain and may cause a clinically apparent and self-limited aseptic meningitis. The patients have an influenzalike illness with headache and photophobia. The cerebrospinal fluid has a pleocytosis, with an increase in cellularity, 20 to 300 cells/µL (normal, 0–5 cells/µL), and an increase in protein to 0.5 to 1.0 g/L. This acute illness is associated with seroconversion to HIV.

Afterward, a slow and progressive subacute encephalitis develops, which is called AIDS encephalopathy or AIDS dementia complex.[187] Early in the disease process the patient will have forgetfulness, slowed thought, and a loss of concentration often associated with depression, apathy, and social withdrawal. This neurologic dysfunction evolves in months to years after the initial HIV infection.

Later, further global deterioration of cognitive function occurs, including motor dysfunction with psychomotor slowing, ataxia, weakness, tremor, incontinence, or psychiatric disturbances.

Late in the disease, the cerebrospinal fluid is also abnormal with an increase in cellularity. Computed tomographic scans of the brain show brain atrophy. The electroencephalography has generalized slowing. At autopsy, the brain is atrophied. Histologically in most cases, there is gliosis of the cerebral cortex with tissue necrosis and microglial nodules. Fewer brains show demyelination, perivascular inflammation, axonal spheroids, and leptomeningeal inflammation. In general, the severity of the histopathologic lesions correlates with the clinical encephalopathy.[185-187]

In addition to the central nervous system involvement, myelopathy and peripheral neuropathies are noted. Patients have progressive spastic paresis and gait ataxia often associated with vacuolar degeneration of the white matter in the spinal cord. A distal symmetric polyneuropathy with numbness, parasthesias, and autonomic dysfunction often occur. Histologically, demyelination, axonopathy, and mononuclear cell infiltrates are noted.[186]

A characteristic feature of AIDS is progressive weight loss and persistent diarrhea. Patients have anorexia and abnormal carbohydrate and fat metabolism. Diarrhea is frequently due to infection.[188] Patients may have gastrointestinal infections with cryptosporidiosis, isosporidia, microsporidia, herpesvirus, cytomegalovirus, and *Mycobacterium avium-intracellulare.*

Kaposi's sarcoma involves the gastrointestinal tract. The cancer is seen in the oropharynx and in the intestines and may be accompanied by a protein-losing enteropathy, bleeding, and bowel perforation.[188]

A variety of hematologic abnormalities are found in individuals with AIDS.[189,190] The blood cell counts are frequently abnormal with anemia, granulocytopenia, and thrombocytopenia. Laboratory tests show anemia of chronic disease, with an increase in ferritin, a low serum iron level, and decreased transferrin. Results of the bone marrow examination often are abnormal with hypercellularity and dysplasia of the hematopoietic cells. These findings may be a consequence of direct infection of the marrow precursor cells with HIV. In addition there are abnormalities of the marrow's lymphoid population, including lymphocytosis and plasmacytosis, which are associated with hypergammaglobulinemia and Coombs'-positive anemia. If lymphoma has developed in the patient, it frequently involves the bone marrow. Granulomas are found, as is marrow necrosis and serous atrophy.[189,190]

Various rheumatologic complications of AIDS occur.[191] Coagulation studies are abnormal in 45% of patients because of a circulating lupus anticoagulant, which causes prolongation of test times in the laboratory but is not associated with bleeding abnormalities. Frequently an anticardiolipin antibody or other autoantibodies, such as antinuclear antibody, antiplatelet antibodies, and anti-RBC antibodies, contribute to the pancytopenia. Symptoms of rheumatologic diseases are found, including oligoarthritis, sacroiliitis, urethritis, and conjunctivitis.[191]

Congestive heart failure develops in some patients with AIDS[192] but is not a common cause of death. There may be cardiac dysfunction related to myocarditis or nonthrombotic endocarditis. Pericarditis and pericardial effusions may occur. Systemic infectious diseases may involve the heart with bacterial endocarditis or bacterial or fungal abscesses in the myocardium. Toxoplasmosis myocarditis occurs rarely.

The kidney is not a target organ in HIV infection, but renal disease may occur.[193] Proteinuria is associated with focal and segmental glomerulosclerosis. This disease progresses to renal failure more rapidly in patients with AIDS than in others. There may be nephrotic syndromes and reflux nephropathy. The kidney may be infected with *Mycobacterium, Cryptococcus,* and cytomegalovirus. Drugs used to treat infection may damage the kidney.[193] Malignancy in patients with AIDS may involve the kidneys.

In the early days of AIDS, unusual skin lesions alerted physicians to the possibility of a new disease.[151] Kaposi's sarcoma was a rare vascular tumor in Europe and North America but was seen more frequently in Africa. In classic Kaposi's sarcoma, the lesions begin on the hands and feet of older men and the progression of the disease is indolent. The AIDS-associated Kaposi's sarcoma is a more aggressive tumor that involves the oral cavity and frequently metastasizes to the lymph nodes, liver, lung, and gastrointestinal system.[151] The disease often pursues a rapidly fatal course.

Skin infections are also commonly seen in patients with AIDS.[194] Molluscum contagiosum is caused by a poxvirus and often leads to papules on the face. Common warts, also called verruca vulgaris, caused by human papillomavirus, occur in patients with AIDS. Herpes zoster infections have occurred, and herpes simplex infections frequently present as severe and chronic perianal ulcerations. Fungal infections with *Cryptococcus* or *Histoplasma* frequently involve the skin, as does infection with *Mycobacterium.*

Most of the cases of AIDS in the United States reported to the CDC are in adult men. Women acquire the disease by intravenous drug abuse or heterosexual encounters with an infected man. In Africa, the rate of female infection is greater, and in areas with high seroprevalence the male-to-female seropositivity approaches 1:1. In addition to the infections, diseases, and other complications already described, women with AIDS have other problems.[195]

Women with AIDS are often in their childbearing years, and fertility is unaffected by HIV infections.[195,196] Normally in pregnancy, women have a physiologic immunosuppression to tolerate the fetus as an allograph. Normal pregnancy is associated with a decrease in the T-cell helper-to-suppressor ratio, T4:T8. The normal lymphoproliferative response to viruses, such as CMV, varicella, herpes, and rubella, decreases.

Pregnant HIV-infected women have an accelerated course from asymptomatic to symptomatic disease. Their disease progresses more rapidly than in HIV-infected male drug users or hemophiliacs.[195] The risk of infections in pregnancy is related to the decrease in number of helper T cells. Pregnancy outcome is adversely affected by HIV in asymptomatic mothers. The incidence of premature rupture of amniotic membranes with preterm labor increases, and more infants are born with a low birth weight.[196]

Perinatal transmission of HIV infection occurs in 33% to 50% of children born to HIV-infected mothers.[196] In areas endemic for HIV infection, seropositivity of cord blood is as high as 2%. The rate of congenital infection with HIV is significantly higher than other congenital viral infections due to CMV, herpesvirus, or rubella.[195] Infection of the fetus occurs early in pregnancy, so delivery by cesarean section is not protective. HIV is secreted in breast milk, and the breast feeding of infants born to HIV-positive mothers is not recommended in the United States. After delivery, HIV-positive women need to have continued medical care for the detection and treatment of opportunistic infections and sexually transmitted disease. Prevention of the immunosuppression of pregnancy in HIV-infected women may require sterilization or abortion.[195,196]

More than 80% of children with HIV are infected before birth. Other children have acquired HIV by the transfusion of blood or blood products.[197] Many infants with congenital HIV infection become symptomatic in the first 18 months of life. Children who have transfusion-related HIV infections become symptomatic more rapidly than adults with posttransfusion HIV. They may have nonspecific symptoms of lymphadenopathy, hepatosplenomegaly, diarrhea, and fever. They fail to gain normal weight and have developmental delays.[197] Children with AIDS have infections caused by bacteria: *Streptococcus pneumoniae, Haemophilus influenzae, Staphylococcus,* and gram-negative species. They have bacterial pneumonia, septicemia, meningitis, cellulitis, and abscesses. They also become infected with opportunistic organisms such as *Pneumocystis*, *Candida*, CMV, *Mycobacterium*, and herpesvirus. Other childhood viral diseases caused by varicella, herpes zoster, rubeola, and EBV may be more severe in the HIV-infected child.[197,198]

In addition to pneumonia, children may develop a noninfectious pulmonary lymphoid hyperplasia. They are hypoxic with chronic interstitial disease. Lymphoid malignancies occur less frequently in children, but polyclonal proliferative lesions are seen. The nervous system is usually involved in the disease process. Children with AIDS exhibit developmental delays or deterioration of their development. Their motor skills, intellect, and behavior are abnormal. They have encephalopathy with paresis, ataxia, and palsy. Their brains are small with inflammatory and histologic abnormalities.[197,198]

Children who have *Pneumocystis* pneumonia in the first year of life have a more rapid clinical course and die by the second birthday. Others may have anti-HIV antibodies and HIV antigens but have a milder clinical course. The degree of immune dysfunction is prognostic.[198,199]

### Typical Disease in the Transfused Individual

HIV contaminated the nation's blood supply in the late 1970s. Cases of transfusion-acquired AIDS (TAA) were reported to the CDC in the early 1980s.[200] Transfusion-acquired AIDS is both similar and dissimilar to AIDS acquired by other infectious routes.

The progression of the disease from asymptomatic carrier to the AIDS-related complex to frank AIDS occurs in TAA. Those transfusion recipients who seroconvert with antibodies to HIV early after transfusion show the AIDS-related conditions more rapidly than those who remain seronegative for more prolonged periods of time. Hemophiliacs who were treated with factor VIII concentrate and had early seroconversion had more lymphadenopathy and lower helper T-cell counts than those who converted late.[201]

Those with TAA had similar immunocompromise and similar opportunistic infections as other patients with AIDS. Children with TAA had *Pneumocystis carinii* pneumonia; adults had Kaposi's sarcoma and opportunistic infections. The mortality rate of TAA as reported by the CDC is high, greater than 50%.[200]

It is not clear whether the disease of AIDS develops more rapidly or is more lethal in those who acquire HIV by transfusion, but a clear difference in TAA is the high rates of infection following exposure. For comparison, heterosexual rates of male-to-female HIV transmission is less than 20%.[202] Congenital infection rates are 33% to 50%.[195,196] Homosexual partners of men with AIDS have a seroconversion rate of 25%.[203]

The risk of HIV infection from blood donors with the virus is great. One study tracing blood recipients of HIV-infected blood found that 59 of 59 patients (100%) were infected, 85% had AIDS, and 15% were carriers.[205] Another report showed that 12 of 12 (100%) neonates developed laboratory or clinical evidence of HIV infection after receiving transfusion of infected blood.[206] A third study gave an infection rate of 62% following the transfusion of blood with HIV.[207] The higher risk may relate to the larger amount of viral inoculum in blood transfusion.

The CDC has collected reports of transfusion-acquired AIDS in the United States. They have found that infants make up a higher proportion of TAA (10% of the total) than would be expected from the numbers of units of blood they receive (2% of the total). The elderly, those older than 70 years of age, had fewer reported cases of transfusion-acquired AIDS than would be expected from the number of transfusions. This might represent a decreased susceptibility to the virus. Alternatively, it might instead be that the elderly who are ill and receive blood transfusions are dying of the underlying disease before the HIV infection becomes symptomatic.[200]

During the past several years, a few sporadic cases have appeared of a disease that is clinically indistinguishable from AIDS but that lacks viral markers or a culturable virus.[244-247] In 2 recent reports,[248,249] the CDC released detailed information on 5 of 26 such cases reported in the literature, together with some general comments on others of the 26 reported at different times.

Each of the patients described in one report[248] were found to have developed a persistently low CD4+ T-lymphocyte count after a variety of pre-existing illnesses. Ultimately, none of these patients recovered from their illnesses. Of the 5 patients described, 2 received transfusion of blood products. Tracing and re-examining of the donors reveal no high-risk behaviors, no suggestive medical history, and complete negativity for all required viral markers. These 5 patients had the following in common: a persistently low CD4+ T-lymphocyte count; clinical features that would lead to the consideration of HIV infection as a differential diagnosis; and the complete absence of viral markers for HIV. In addition, clinical recovery was noted.

As of August 1992, the CDC has received reports of 9 additional such cases in the United States.[249] All of these cases meet the criteria for an apparently new entity: CD4+ T-cell lymphopenia without evidence of HIV infection (documented CD4+ count of <300 cells/μL or <0% on more than 1 occasion; negative laboratory evidence of HIV markers, including antibody testing, p24 antigen detection, polymerase chain reaction, and viral culture; and no apparent immunodeficiency correlative with the depressed CD4+ levels).

Concern has been expressed, both in the United States and at the recent International Conference on AIDS (Paris, July 1992), that some of these cases might be attributable to another retroviral agent, undetectable by current technologies. The patients described in detail in this country appear to undergo clinical recovery. Furthermore, no viral agent is yet attributable to the retrovirus series found in association with them, no linkage with blood transfusion can be associated, and these cases are rare. A general consensus appears to be developing that it is unlikely that such cases pose any real threat to the nation's blood supply. To be sure, further investigations are essential and are being conducted now. Interim reports will be issued at frequent intervals by the CDC as the studies progress. It seems exceedingly unlikely, however, that the occurrence of such cases will contribute in any way to a risk of transfusion-transmissible disease.

As of August 1992, the risk of viral transmission by blood products appears to be further receding. For example, the per-unit risk for HIV is 1 in 225,000, and significant improvements in hepatitis risk can also be demonstrated.[250] It is probably accurate to state that, at the present time, the blood supply of the nation is safer than it has ever been before.[250]

## Steps Taken to Minimize the Risks

In the 1990s, individuals whose behaviors put them at risk for AIDS are not allowed to donate blood. All blood products are tested for antibody to HIV. The risk of HIV transmission by blood products has been greatly reduced.[162,163] For hemophiliacs, factor VIII concentrate treated to inactivate viruses is now available.[208]

### Infectivity of Blood Products

Before serologic tests for anti-HIV antibody were available, blood products that transmitted AIDS included packed RBCs, platelets, plasma, and whole blood.[200] Factor VIII hemophiliacs and those with von Willebrand's disease who have received factor VIII concentrates have acquired AIDS, as have factor IX hemophiliacs who have received factor IX concentrates. Products prepared before donor self-exclusions and HIV antibody screening in the mid 1980s have a greater risk of transmitting AIDS.

Blood collected from donors who have the virus but have not developed antibody may still be infectious. The risk of this occurring has been estimated to be from 1:28,000 in a multiply transfused patient to 1:153,000 for a single-unit recipient.[162,163]

## BACTERIA

Donor blood is drawn, tested, and stored in the blood bank for administration to a patient. At each step, techniques are used to prevent the contamination of the blood with bacteria. However, fatalities caused by septic shock have been and continue to be reported as untoward consequences of bacterial contamination of banked blood.[209-211]

### Microbiology

The bacteria that have been reported to cause transfusion reactions are listed in Table 3-1. Gram-negative bacteria have caused the most fatal transfusion reactions. These strains proliferate at blood storage temperatures and, following transfusion, have induced septic shock.[212]

**TABLE 3-1** **BACTERIA THAT HAVE BEEN REPORTED IN TRANSFUSION REACTIONS [221-230]**

| | |
|---|---|
| *Achromobacter* | Anaerobic bacilli |
| *Paracolobactrum aerogenoides* | Gram-positive bacilli |
| *Escherichia coli* | *Staphylococcus albus* |
| *Pseudomonas* | *Staphylococcus epidermidis* |
| *Aerobacter* | Gram-positive anaerobic cocci |
| *Alcaligenes faecalis* | Hemolytic colli |
| Brucellosis | |
| *Yersinia* | |

## Typical Disease in the Nontransfused Individual

Septic shock has been defined as circulatory failure following exposure to microbial toxins.[213] Most cases of septic shock are caused by gram-negative bacilli (Table 3-2), but shock has also been seen complicating infections with gram-positive microorganisms, rickettsia, fungi, and viruses.[214-218]

**TABLE 3-2** | **BACTERIA COMMONLY ASSOCIATED WITH SEPTIC SHOCK**[226,227]

| | |
|---|---|
| *Escherichia coli* | *Klebsiella* |
| *Enterobacter* | *Serratia* |
| *Pseudomonas* | *Proteus* |
| *Providencia* | *Bacteroides* |

Bacteremia, or the presence of bacteria in the blood, is not synonymous with septicemia, the disease associated with microorganisms or their toxins in the blood. Transient bacteremia is a common condition that has been caused by activities such as toothbrushing and dental flossing and occurs following minor operative procedures such as dental extractions, sigmoidoscopy, and liver biopsy.[219] Ordinarily, the bacteria are rapidly cleared by the reticuloendothelial cells, such as Kupffer's cells in the liver, or phagocytized by neutrophils in the circulation. Only about 30% of hospitalized patients with bacteremia develop sepsis.

When bacteremia occurs in a compromised individual (one who is elderly, malnourished, or debilitated) disease may follow.[220] Those who have cancer, chronic diseases of the heart, liver, or kidneys, or conditions such as alcoholism or diabetes mellitus are at risk for septicemia. Patients who are immunosuppressed or have undergone trauma or surgical procedures have increased risk for sepsis.[220]

Septic shock is defined as the circulatory failure that follows the host's response to microbes or microbial toxins. The microbes are usually gram-negative bacteria that invade from the genitourinary tract, gastrointestinal tract, lung, or skin. The response to the bacteremia is circulatory failure. A result is that systemic tissue perfusion is inadequate. In the beginning the cardiac output and blood pressure are normal,[213,214] but peripheral venous pooling occurs. The decreased venous return leads to a decrease in cardiac output. The decrease in cardiac output further decreases perfusion of tissues, resulting in acidosis. The blood pressure decreases, and urinary output is reduced. Shock may progress with pulmonary, cardiac, and renal failure and death.

The clinical management of septic shock is aimed at treating the underlying infection with appropriate antibiotics and therapeutic intervention.[215] To support the cardiovascular circulation, intravascular volume is increased with intravenous fluids. Inotropic agents such as dopamine or dobutamine are used to maintain blood pressure. Mechanical ventilation will decrease the work of breathing, support the heart, and treat metabolic acidosis.

The outcome of the shock varies with underlying condition of the patient. Of those patients with septic shock, 30% to 80% die. The more ill and debilitated the patient was before the septic shock occurs, the greater the possibility of mortality. The source of the infection must be identified and appropriate antibiotics must be used.

### Typical Disease in the Transfused Individual

The infusion of blood contaminated with bacteria has a characteristic clinical syndrome. The patient has a violent chill as the unit runs in or shortly thereafter,[220] while exhibiting symptoms of fever, tachycardia, hypotension, nausea, vomiting, and circulatory collapse. This reaction is distinguished from a hemolytic transfusion reaction by a lack of hemoglobinemia or hemoglobinuria. Many of those described to have posttransfusion septic shock have died.[209-212,218] Survival depends on the recognition of septic shock, discontinuation of the infusion, and the institution of appropriate antibiotic drugs and supportive measures. As with septic shock in other clinical settings, the more compromised the patient is from the underlying disease, the greater the risk of death.

### Steps Taken to Minimize the Risks

Each step of blood collection, storage, and transfusion must be carefully monitored to prevent the introduction of bacteria into the unit and to prevent the contaminant from proliferating. The donor evaluation is designed to screen out those who may have bacteremia. Blood from donors with acute illness (cough, diarrhea, bronchitis, colds, influenza, sore throats, or skin lesions) is not drawn.[221] Donors who appear ill or who have abnormal temperatures or heart or respiratory rates are deferred. Since bacteremia is reported to follow dental work,[219] donors are asked to refrain from donating until 72 hours after their dental visit. Despite these measures some units are drawn while the donor is having an episode of bacteremia.[220]

Bacteria may be introduced into the donated blood as the unit is drawn. To minimize this risk the skin is carefully cleansed with soap, alcohol, and iodine. The needle is pushed into the vein with care not to cut a core of skin. Bacteria deep in pores are not removed by cleansing the surface. A core of skin introduced into the bag may carry surface contaminants.

The unit is drawn into a sterile bag with sterile anticoagulant. In the early days of blood banking, sterilized glass bottles were used. This procedure increased the risk for bacteria to be drawn into the bottle as it was vented. These bottles also had to be physically entered to withdraw blood for testing or to prepare pooled products.

Tests on blood units drawn into bottles in the 1950s showed a 2% contamination rate. Most bacteria cultured from these units (95%) were *Staphylococcus,* an organism that has not caused fatal transfusion reactions.[216] The closed plastic units currently used have less risk for bacterial contamination.

Blood has some inherent capabilities for killing bacteria or preventing their growth.[216] Freshly drawn blood contains polymorphonuclear leukocytes and monocytes that phagocytize bacteria. The anticoagulated plasma contains antibacterial antibodies and complement to further suppress bacterial proliferation. In addition, studies of bacterial growth at room temperature show that when bacteria are deliberately introduced, bacterial proliferation does not begin immediately but is delayed for 4 to 6 hours.[216]

Donor blood is immediately refrigerated and is kept refrigerated in storage. The refrigerators in the blood bank are monitored to ensure that the 4°C temperature is maintained. When blood is taken to the ward, but not used, the unit must be returned within 30 minutes, which ensures that the temperature does not rise above 6°C. It is recommended that units be promptly hung and infused.

Platelets have a different storage than other blood products. Pooled platelets are kept at room temperature, 22°C, for 72 hours. Studies have determined that platelets can be drawn and prepared in a sterile manner.[222] When bacteria are deliberately inoculated into platelet packs, leukocytes will kill the bacteria and inhibit bacterial growth. Like blood, platelets stored in plasma with neutrophils have bactericidal and bacteriostatic properties.[222]

In the blood bank, care is taken not to inoculate bacteria in the stored units. The blood is stored in bags with small samples of blood available for testing without requiring that the unit be opened. When a bag is opened to wash the blood or to draw off smaller amounts for transfusion, the unit must be discarded after 24 hours. This rule further protects blood recipients from possible bacterial septicemia.

Before blood is administered, it is visually inspected. Proliferation of gram-negative bacteria often causes the blood cells to lyse, and free hemoglobin will be visible in plasma. Gram-negative bacteria may metabolize the citrate in the blood unit; the citrate is added as an anticoagulant. The liberation of calcium from the metabolized citrate may induce clotting of the blood in the unit. Blood clotting will be visualized as clumped or congealed blood. These units are not used but discarded.[221]

### Infectivity of Blood Products

Septicemia has occurred following the transfusion of blood, plasma, and cryoprecipitate.[211]

## Syphilis

In the early days of blood transfusion, when donor blood was directly transmitted without storage in a blood bank, syphilis was a recognized posttransfusion infection.[223,224] The infectiousness of donor blood has been limited by serologic screening and ordinary storage techniques.[224]

### Microbiology

*Treponema pallidum* is a spirochete responsible for the sexually transmitted disease, syphilis. *Treponema* spirochetes also cause other diseases: *T. pallidum* subspecies *pertenue* causes yaws; *T. pallidum* subspecies *endemicum* causes nonvenereal syphilis; and *T. carateum* causes pinta.[225] *Treponema* species have not been cultured to allow detailed microbiologic studies.

### Typical Disease in the Nontransfused Individual

Nearly all cases of syphilis are acquired by sexual contact. The organism penetrates mucous membranes to produce a primary lesion, the chancre at the site of entry as well as proliferation in the systemic circulation. Six to 8 weeks later, secondary skin lesions occur, with generalized lymph edema. Hepatitis and glomerulonephritis may develop, and the host may be infectious for 24 years. Antibodies develop to *Treponema*.

If untreated, a progression inflammatory disease begins, including syphilitic aortitis and neurosyphilis. Syphilis occurs with endarteritis of vessels in the vasorum of the aorta, which produces medial necrosis of the vessel with destruction of elastic tissue. An aneurysm of the aorta is formed with associated aortic regurgitation or coronary ostia stenosis. These cardiovascular abnormalities may cause premature death. Infection of the central nervous system (CNS) leads to chronic disease in many untreated individuals. Symptomatic neurosyphilis occurs with premature stroke, paresis, tabes dorsalis, and optic atrophy. These complications are prevented by early diagnosis and treatment.[225]

### Typical Disease in the Transfused Individual

Following transfusion of infected donor blood, the recipient weeks later may show signs of secondary syphilis (rash and fever). If untreated the disease may progress.

### Infectivity of Blood Products

Syphilis has been transmitted in fresh whole blood.[223,224] Fresh or frozen plasma may also transmit the infection.[226]

### Steps Taken to Minimize the Risks

Donors are initially screened by history to eliminate those with venereal infections. Blood from those with open sores is not drawn. After blood donation, units are tested for serologic evidence of *T. pallidum* exposure, and positive units are discarded. The storage and refrigeration of blood at 4°C for 48 to 96 hours eliminates its infectivity.[227]

## MALARIA

Malaria, a protozoan disease, is usually transmitted to humans by the bite of the *Anopheles* mosquito,[228] but it may be accidentally transmitted by the transfusion of blood.[229] This complication, transfusion-induced malaria, is rare in the United States because malaria is no longer an indigenous disease. It has occurred following the donation of blood from donors who have lived or traveled in endemic areas. The American Association of Blood Banks has guidelines to restrict the donation of blood from individuals who have had malaria or who have traveled in endemic areas.[230]

### Biologic Characteristics

The causative agents of malaria are protozoa of the genus *Plasmodium*. Malaria is transmitted by the *Anopheles* mosquito as it feeds. Malaria sporozoites in the mosquito salivary gland gain access into humans[231] and migrate in the peripheral blood to the liver. The sporozoites in hepatocytes undergo asexual multiplication to form merozoites. The merozoites escape into the circulation and infect RBCs.

The parasite initially appears as a ring-shaped triphozite in the RBCs and divides to form a schizont. After 48 to 72 hours the erythrocyte ruptures, releasing new merozoites, each of which is capable of infecting another RBC.[231] After a few cycles, the merozoites form the sexually active forms, the gametocytes.

The RBCs with gametocytes do not rupture but await entry into a feeding mosquito. The gametocytes undergo fertilization in the gut of the mosquito and multiply to form sporozoites. The sporozoites migrate to the salivary gland, to await another cycle of infection.[228]

### Typical Disease in the Nontransfused Individual

The symptoms of malaria are caused by the rupture of infected erythrocytes to release merozoites. Patients have fever and chills in 48- or 72-hour intervals and become anemic due to the destruction of RBCs. Severe intravascular hemolysis may occur with marked anemia, hemoglobinemia, and hemoglobinuria. Hypoxia leads to renal tubular necrosis and hepatic centrilobular necrosis. Congestive heart failure may be related to the increased work of the heart caused by anemia. Pulmonary edema, hypersplenism, and disseminated intravascular coagulation are sometimes seen.[232]

Infections with some species of *Plasmodium,* including *P. vivax, P. ovale,* and *P. malariae,* are generally not life-threatening and may resolve clinically without specific therapy after several febrile cycles. *Plasmodium falciparum* may cause severe illness and death. Cerebral anoxia may cause disorientation, psychosis, and coma. Seizures are frequent. A poor prognosis is seen in patients with a high density of parasites and severe anemia. Pregnant women, young children, and the elderly have an increased risk of complications when parasitemia is high; survival is dependent on antimalarial drugs and supportive medical care.[231,232]

### Typical Disease in the Transfused Individual

The disease seen in posttransfusion malaria is similar to that in acquired malaria. The period from incubation to onset of symptoms varies with the parasitic load. Deaths have occurred in transfused individuals.[229,233,234]

### Steps Taken to Minimize the Risks

Questions in the donor history are designed to detect travel in areas in which malaria is endemic. Those travelers who have not taken prophylactic antimalarial medication and have not developed malaria may donate blood 6 months after their return. Donors who have taken antimalarial medication are deferred for 3 years after their return from endemic areas. Donors who have had malaria are deferred for 3 years after the cessation of therapy if they have been asymptomatic. No screening test is used to evaluate donor units for malaria.[230]

## Babesiosis

Babesiosis is a rarely occurring disease in humans that is caused by the intracellular erythrocyte parasite, *Babesia microti.* Just as malaria has been transmitted by transfused blood, babesiosis has been transmitted by blood products in areas where the infection is endemic.

### Microbiology

Babesiosis is a tick-transmitted disease of a malarialike erythrocyte parasite.[235] About 20 species of *Babesia* infect many species of mammals, including domesticated animals and wild rodents. In animals, the virulence of the infections varies from lethal to mildly symptomatic. Human infections are uncommon.

The disease is transmitted by hard-bodied ticks, the family Ixodidae, while the tick feeds on the mammalian host.[236] The ticks are infected by 2 mechanisms: by feeding on infected mammals and by transovarian infection of developing embryos. The parasite lives in the salivary gland of the tick.

*Babesia* organisms invade erythrocytes, grow, and multiply. The parasitic forms are irregular: they may be round, rod-shaped, pyriform, or ameboid. They multiply in the RBCs. The RBCs lyse with resultant anemia, hemoglobinuria, and bilirubinemia.

### Typical Disease in the Nontransfused Individual

Babesiosis is a zoonosis transmitted in humans by hard-bodied ticks of the Ixodidae family. Parasitemia is sometimes asymptomatic or subclinical, and the diagnosis is made retrospectively by serologic studies.[237] Infected, symptomatic patients have a mild-to-moderate hemolytic anemia with fever, chills and sweats, myalgia, arthralgia, and fatigue.[238] Hemoglobinuria and renal failure may ensue. Patients who have undergone splenectomy have a more severely symptomatic illness, and fatalities have been reported.[239]

### Typical Disease in the Transfused Individual

Human babesiosis is usually transmitted by ticks, but a review of the literature indicates that 14% of cases in 1 series occurred following the transfusion of infected blood products.[240-242] The incubation period is 6 to 8 weeks. The disease in transfused patients is similar to symptomatic disease in others with babesiosis but may be more severe in patients with underlying illness. An elderly patient has died after the transfusion of infected packed RBCs.[242]

### Steps Taken to Minimize the Risks

The reports of babesiosis in the United States are restricted geographically to islands and costal lands of the Northeast: Nantucket Island, Martha's Vineyard, and Cape Cod, Massachusetts, and Long Island, New York.[236-238] Prospective donors in these areas are asked about a history of babesiosis or tick bite and may be deferred from donation.[242]

### Infectivity of Blood Products

Posttransfusion babesiosis has occurred following the transfusion of RBCs, frozen deglycerolized RBCs, and platelets.[235,240,243]

## References


1. Zuckerman AJ. The history of viral hepatitis from antiquity to the present. In: Deinhardt F, Deinhardt J, eds. Viral Hepatitis, Laboratory and Clinical Science. New York, NY: Marcel Dekker; 1983:3.
2. Krugman S. History of acute viral hepatitis. In Gitnick G, ed. Modern Concepts of Acute and Chronic Hepatitis. New York, NY: Plenum Medical Book Co; 1989:3.
3. Dean JA, Ognibene AJ. Hepatitis in Medical Department, United States Army in Vietnam. Internal Medicine in Vietnam. Washington, DC: US Government Printing Office; 1982;2:419.
4. Blumer G. Infectious jaundice in the United States. JAMA. 1923;81:353.
5. Beeson PB. Jaundice occurring one to four months after transfusion of blood or plasma. JAMA. 1949;121:1332.
6. Neefe JR, Stokes J, Gellis SS. Homologous serum hepatitis and infectious (epidemic) hepatitis. Am J Med Sci. 1945;210:561.
7. Krugman S, Giles JP, Hammond J. Infectious hepatitis: evidence for two distinctive clinical, epidemiologic and immunologic types of infection. JAMA. 1967;200:365.
8. Blumberg BS, Alter HJ, Visnich S. Australian antigen: a new antigen in leukemic sera. JAMA. 1965;191:541.
9. Prince AM. An antigen detected in the blood during the incubation period of serum hepatitis. Proc Natl Acad Sci. 1968;60:814.
10. Koretz RL. Prognosis of acute viral hepatitis. In: Gitnick G, ed. Modern Concepts of Acute and Chronic Hepatitis. New York, NY: Plenum Medical Book Co; 1989.
11. Gerber MA, Thung SN. Biology of disease: molecular and cellular pathology of hepatitis B. Lab Invest. 1985;52:572.
12. Feinstone SM, Kapikian AZ, Purcell RH. Hepatitis A: detection by immune electron microscopy of a virus-like antigen associated with acute illness. Science. 1973;182:1026.
13. Provost PJ, Ittensofin OL, Villarejos VM, Hilleman MR. A specific complement-fixation test for human hepatitis A. Proc Soc Exp Biol Med. 1975;148:961.
14. Ticehurst JR, Racaniello VR, Baroudy BM, et al. Molecular cloning and characterization of hepatitis A viral cDNA. Proc Natl Acad Sci. 1983;80:5885.
15. Siegl G. The biochemistry of hepatitis A virus. In: Gerety RJ, ed. Hepatitis A. New York, NY: Academic Press; 1984:9-32.
16. Aach RD, Kahn RA. Post-transfusion hepatitis, current perspectives. Ann Intern Med. 1980;92:539.
17. Seeberg S, Brandberg A, Hermodsson S, et al. Hospital outbreak of hepatitis A secondary to blood exchange in a baby. Lancet. 1981;1:1155.
18. Hollinger FB, Khan NC, Definger PE, et al. Post-transfusion hepatitis type A. JAMA. 1983;250:2313.
19. Noble RC, Kane MA, Reeves SA, Roeckel I. Post-transfusion hepatitis A in a neonatal intensive care unit. JAMA. 1984;252:2711.
20. Hadler SC, Margolis HS. Viral hepatitis. In: Evans AS, ed. Viral Infections of Humans: Epidemiology and Control. 3rd ed. New York, NY: Plenum Medical Book Co; 1989:351-391.
21. Melnick JL. Enteroviruses. In: Evans AS, ed. Viral Infections of Humans: Epidemiology & Control. 3rd ed. New York, NY: Plenum Medical Book Co; 1989:191-264.
22. Feinstone SM, Gust TD. Modern concepts of hepatitis A. In Gitnick G, ed. Modern Concepts of Acute and Chronic Hepatitis. New York, NY: Plenum Medical Book Co; 1989.

23. Lemon SM. Type A viral hepatitis. N Engl J Med. 1985;313:1059.
24. Ruekert RR. Picornaviruses and their replication. In Fields BN, ed. Fundamental Virology. New York, NY: Raven Press; 1988:357-390.
25. Cohen JL, Ticehurst JR, Purcell RH, et al. Complete nucleotide sequence of wild type hepatitis A virus: comparison with different strains of hepatitis A virus and other picornaviruses. J Virol. 1987;61:50.
26. Francis DP, Hadler SC, Prendergast TJ, et al. Occurrence of hepatitis A, B, and non-A/non-B in the United States. Am J Med. 1984;76:69.
27. Hadler SC, McFarland L. Hepatitis in daycare centers: epidemiology and prevention. Rev Infect Dis. 1986;8:548.
28. Corey L, Holmes KK. Sexual transmission of hepatitis A in homosexual men. N Engl J Med. 1980;307:435.
29. Junge LL, Deinhardt FT. The acute manifestations of hepatitis B virus infection. In Gerety RJ, ed. Hepatitis B. Orlando, Fla: Academic Press; 1985:94-118.
30. Gordon SC, Reddy KR, Schiff L, Schiff ER. Prolonged intrahepatic cholestasis secondary to acute hepatitis A. Ann Intern Med. 1984;101:635.
31. Dodolsky DR, Isselbacher KJ. Hepatic encephaly. In Braunwald E, ed. Harrison's Principles of Internal Medicine. 11th ed. New York, NY: McGraw-Hill Book Co; 1987:1349-1350.
32. Tabor E. Clinical presentation of hepatitis A. In Gerety RJ, ed. Hepatitis A. Orlando, Fla: Academic Press; 1984:47-54.
33. Wollheim FA. Immunoglobulins in the course of viral hepatitis, and in cholestatic and obstructive jaundice. Acta Med Scand. 1968;183:473.
34. Purcell RH, Wong DC, Moritsugu Y, et al. A microtiter solid-phase radioimmunoassay for hepatitis A antigen and antibody. J Immunol. 1976;116:349.
35. Lemon SM, Brown CD, Brooks DS, et al. Specific immunoglobulin in response to hepatitis A virus determined by solid-phase radioimmunoassay. Infect Immun. 1980;28:927.
36. Villarejos VM, Serra JC, Anderson-Visona K, Mosley JW. Hepatitis A virus infection in households. Am J Epidemiol. 1982;115:577.
37. Ticehurst JR, Feinstone SM, Chestnut T, et al. Detection of hepatitis A virus by extraction of viral RNA and molecular hybridization. J Clin Microbiol. 1987;25:1822.
38. Blum HE, Vyas GN. Non-A, non-B hepatitis: a contemporary assessment. Haematology. 1982;15:162.
39. Barbara JA, Howell DR, Briggs M, Parry JV. Post-transfusion hepatitis A. Lancet. 1982;1:738.
40. Werner BG, Grady GF. Hepatitis prophylaxis. In: Gitnick G, ed. Modern Concepts of Acute and Chronic Hepatitis. New York, NY: Plenum Medical Book Co; 1989:188-189.
41. Morgon HV, Williamson DAJ. Jaundice following administration of human blood products. Br Med J. 1943;1:750.
42. Bigger JW. Jaundice in syphilitics under treatment. Lancet. 1943;1:457.
43. Goldfield M. Some epidemiologic studies of transfusion-associated hepatitis. In Greenwalt TJ, Jamieson GA, eds. Transmissible Disease and Blood Transfusion. New York, NY: Grune & Stratton; 1974:141-151.
44. Alter HJ, Holland PV, Purcell RH, et al. Post-transfusion hepatitis after exclusion of commercial and hepatitis-B antigen donors. Ann Intern Med. 1972;77:691.
45. Knodell RG, Conrad ME, Dienstag JL, Bell CJ. Etiological spectrum of post-transfusion hepatitis. Gastroenterology. 1975;69:1278.
46. Driss F, Bobac B, Zarski JP, et al. An epidemiological and clinical study of transaminase levels and hepatitis B antibodies in 1,100 blood donors. Vox Sang. 1989;57:43.
47. Galibert F, Mandart E, Fitoussi F, et al. Nucleotide sequence of the hepatitis B virus genome. Nature. 1979;281:646.

48. Gerber MA, Thung SN. Pathobiology of hepatitis B virus. Pathobiol Ann. 1981;11:197.
49. Dane DS, Cameron CH, Briggs M. Virus-like particles in serum of some patients with Australia antigen associated hepatitis. Lancet. 1970;1:695.
50. Alter MJ, Hadler SC, Margolis HS, Alexander WJ. The changing epidemiology of hepatitis B in the United States. JAMA. 1990;263:1218.
51. Krugman S, Overby LR, Mushahwar IK, et al. Viral hepatitis, type B, studies on natural history and prevention re-examined. N Engl J Med. 1979;300:101.
52. Inman RD, McDougal JS, Redecha PB, et al. Isolation and characterization of circulating immune complexes in patients with hepatitis B systemic vasculitis. Clin Immunol Immunopathol. 1981;21:364.
53. Brechot C, Degos F, Lugassy C, et al. Hepatitis B virus DNA in patients with chronic liver disease and negative tests for hepatitis B surface antigens. N Engl J Med. 1985;312:270.
54. Feinman SV, Cooter N, Sinclair JC, et al. Clinical and epidemiological significance of HBsAg (Australia antigen): carrier state. Gastroenterology. 1975;68:113.
55. Hoofnagle JH, Seeff LB, Bales ZB, Zimmerman HJ. Type B hepatitis after transfusion with blood containing antibody to hepatitis B core antigen. N Engl J Med. 1978;298:1379.
56. Allen JG, Sayman WA. Serum hepatitis from transfusions of blood. JAMA. 1962;180:1079.
57. Gocke DJ. A prospective study of post-transfusion hepatitis. JAMA. 1972;219:1165.
58. Giusti G, Galanti B, Gaeta GB, Gall C. Etiology, clinical and laboratory data of post-transfusion hepatitis: a retrospective study of 379 cases from 53 Italian hospitals. Infection. 1987;15:111.
59. Grady GF, Chalmers TC, the Boston Inter-Hospital Liver Group. Risk of post-transfusion viral hepatitis. N Engl J Med. 1964;271:337.
60. Walker RH, ed. Technical Manual. 10th ed. Arlington, Va: American Association of Blood Banks; 1990:1-18.
61. Alter HJ, Seeff LB, Kaplan PM, et al. Type B hepatitis: the infectivity of blood positive for e antigen & DNA polymerase after accidental needle stick exposure. N Engl J Med. 1976;295:909.
62. Rizzetto M, Canese MG, Arico S, et al. Immunofluoresence detection of new antigen: antibody system (d/anti d) associated to hepatitis B virus in liver and in serum of HBsAg carriers. Gut. 1977;18:997.
63. Fields HA, Hadler SC. Delta hepatitis: a review. J Clin Immunoassay. 1986;9:128.
64. Ponzetto A, Forzani B, Parravincini P, et al. Epidemiology of hepatitis delta virus (HDV) infection. Eur J Epidemiol. 1985;1:257.
65. Hadler SC, De Monzon M, Ponzetto A, et al. Delta virus infection and severe hepatitis. Ann Intern Med. 1984;100:339.
66. Rosina F, Saracco G, Rizzetto M. Risk of post-transfusion infection with hepatitis delta virus. N Engl J Med. 1985;312:1488.
67. Roche JK, Stengle JM. Comparison of the sensitivities of newer detection systems for hepatitis B antigen. Transfusion. 1973;13:258.
68. Koretz RL, Klahs DR, Ritman S, et al. Posttransfusion hepatitis in recipients of blood screened by newer assays. Lancet. 1973;1:694.
69. Bonino F, Smedile A. Delta agent (type D) hepatitis. Semin Liver Dis. 1986;6:28.
70. Rizzetto M, Morello C, Mannucci PM, et al. Delta infection and liver disease in hemophilic carriers of hepatitis B surface antigen. J Infect Dis. 1981;141:18.
71. Grady GF, Bennett AJE. Risk of post-transfusion hepatitis in the United States. JAMA. 1972;220:692.
72. Gocke DJ, Greenberg HB, Kavey NB. Hepatitis antigen: detection of infectious blood donors. Lancet. 1970;2:248.

73. Hollinger FB, Werch J, Melnick JL. A prospective study indicating that double-antibody radioimmunoassay reduces the incidence of post-transfusion hepatitis B. N Engl J Med. 1974;290:1104.
74. Senior JR, Sutnick AI, Goeser E, et al. Reduction of post-transfusion hepatitis by exclusion of Australia antigen from donor blood in an urban public hospital. Am J Med Sci. 1974;267:171.
75. Alter HJ, Holland PV, Purcell RH. The emerging pattern of post-transfusion hepatitis. Am J Med Sci. 1975;270:329.
76. Hoofnagle JH, Gerety RJ, Tabor E, et al. Transmission of non A, non B hepatitis. Ann Intern Med. 1977;87:14.
77. Mosley JW. Hepatitis types B and non-B. JAMA. 1975;233:967.
78. Mosley JW. The epidemiology of viral hepatitis: an overview. Am J Med Sci. 1975;270:253.
79. Blum HE, Vyas GN. Non-A, non-B hepatitis: a contemporary assessment. Haematologia. 1982;15:153.
80. Alter JH, Purcell RH, Holland PV, et al. Donor transaminase and recipient hepatitis. JAMA. 1981;246:630.
81. Zuck TF, Sherwood WC, Bove JR. A review of recent events related to surrogate testing of blood to prevent non-A, non-B post-transfusion hepatitis. Transfusion. 1987;27:203.
82. Choo QL, Kuo G, Weiner AJ, et al. Isolation of a cDNA clone derived from a blood-borne non-A, non-B viral hepatitis genome. Science. 1989;244:359.
83. Kuo G, Choo QL, Alter HJ, et al. An assay of circulating antibodies to a major etiologic virus of human non-A, non-B hepatitis. Science. 1989;244:362.
84. Roggendorf M, Deinhardt F, Rasshofer R, et al. Antibodies to hepatitis C virus. Lancet. 1989;2:324.
85. Hopf H, Moller B, Kuther D, et al. Long-term follow up of post-transfusion and sporadic chronic hepatitis non-A, non-B and frequency of circulating antibodies to hepatitis C virus (HCV). J Hepatol. 1990;10:69.
86. Rumi MG, Colombo M, Gringeri A, Mannercci PM. High prevalence of antibody to hepatitis C virus in multi-transfused transaminases. Ann Intern Med. 1990;112:379.
87. Miyamura T, Saito Z, Katayama T, et al. Detection of antibody against antigen expressed by molecularly cloned hepatitis C virus cDNA: application to diagnosis and blood screening for posttransfusion hepatitis. Proc Natl Acad Sci. 1990;87:983.
88. Weiner A, et al. Detection of hepatitis C viral sequences in non-A, non-B hepatitis. Lancet. 1990;335:1.
89. He LF, Alling D, Popkin T, et al. Determining the size of non-A, non-B hepatitis virus by filtration. J Infect Dis. 1987;156:636.
90. Miller RH, Purcell RH. Hepatitis C virus shares amino acid sequence similarity with pestivirus and flavivirus as well as members of two plant virus supergroups. Proc Natl Acad Sci. 1990;87:2057.
91. Alter MJ, Coleman PJ, Alexander J, et al. Importance of heterosexual activity in the transmission of hepatitis B and non-A, non-B hepatitis. JAMA. 1989;262:1201.
92. Alter MJ, Hadler SC, Judson FN, et al. Risk factors for acute non-A non-B hepatitis in the United States and association with hepatitis C virus infection. JAMA. 1990;264:2231.
93. Dienstag JL. Non-A, non-B hepatitis, I: recognition, epidemiology and clinical features. Gastroenterology. 1983;85:439.
94. Alter HJ, Prince AM. Transfusion-associated non-A, non-B hepatitis: an assessment of the causative agent and its clinical impact. Transfusion Med Rev. 1988;2:288.
95. Alter HJ, Hoofnagle JH. Non-A, non-B: observations on the first decade. In: Vyas GN, Dienstag JL, Hoofnagle JH, eds. Viral Hepatitis and Liver Disease. New York, NY: Grune & Stratton; 1984:345-354.

96. Aach RD, Szmuness W, Mosley JW, et al. Serum alanine aminotransferase of donors in relation to the risk of non-A non-B hepatitis in recipients. N Engl J Med. 1981;304:989.
97. Stevens CE, Aach RD, Hollinger FB, et al. Hepatitis B virus antibody in blood donors and the occurrence of non-A non-B hepatitis in transfusion recipients. Ann Intern Med. 1984;101:733.
98. Koziol DE, Holland PV, Alling DW, et al. Antibody to hepatitis B core antigen as a paradoxical marker for non-A non-B hepatitis agents in donated blood. Ann Intern Med. 1986;104:488.
99. van der Poel CL, Reesink HW, Schaasberg W, et al. Infectivity of blood seropositive for hepatitis C virus antibodies. Lancet. 1990;335:558.
100. Lang DJ. Transfusion- and perfusion-associated cytomegalovirus and Epstein-Barr virus infections. In: Greenwalt TJ, Jamieson GA, eds. Transmissible Disease and Blood Transfusion. New York, NY: Grune & Stratton; 1974:153-169.
101. Kaariainen L, Klemola E, Paloheimo J. Rise of cytomegalovirus antibodies in an infectious mononucleosis-like syndrome after transfusion. Br Med J. 1966;1:1270.
102. Tegtmeier GE. Post-transfusion cytomegalovirus infections. Arch Pathol Lab Med. 1989;113:236.
103. Roizman B. Herpesviridae: a brief introduction. In: Fields BN, Knipe DM, eds. Virology. 2nd ed. New York, NY: Raven Press; 1990:1787-1793.
104. Stagno S. Cytomegalovirus. In: Remington JS, Klein JO, eds. Infectious Disease of the Fetus and Newborn. 3rd ed. Philadelphia, Pa: WB Saunders; 1990:241-281.
105. Doerr HW. Cytomegalovirus infection in pregnancy. J Virol Methods. 1987;17:127.
106. Yow MD. Congenital cytomegalovirus disease: a new problem. J Infect Dis. 1989;159:163.
107. Macdonald H, Tobin JOH. Congenital cytomegalovirus infection: a collaborative study on epidemiological, clinical and laboratory findings. Dev Med Child Neurol. 1978;20:471.
108. Dudgeon JA. Infective causes of human malformations. Br Med Bull. 1976;32:77.
109. Drew WL. Diagnosis of cytomegalovirus infection. Rev Infect Dis. 1988;10:5468.
110. Demmler GJ, Yow MD, Spector SA, et al. Nosocomial cytomegalovirus infections within two hospitals caring for infants and children. J Infect Dis. 1987;156:9.
111. Hanshaw JB, Betts RF, Simon G, Boynton RC. Acquired cytomegalovirus infection. N Engl J Med. 1965;272:602.
112. Onorato IM, Morens DM, Martone WJ, Stansfield SK. Epidemiology of cytomegalovirus infections. Rev Infect Dis. 1985;7:479.
113. Klemola E, von Essen R, Wager O, et al. Cytomegalovirus mononucleosis in previously healthy individuals. Ann Intern Med. 1969;71:11.
114. Alford CA, Britt WJ. Cytomegalovirus. In: Fields BN, Knipe DM, eds. Virology. 2nd ed. New York, NY: Raven Press; 1990:1981-2010.
115. Jordan MC. Cytomegalovirus infections. In: Hoeprich PD, Jordan MC, eds. Infectious Diseases. 4th ed. Philadelphia, Pa: JB Lippincott; 1989:805-811.
116. Abdallah PS, Mark JBD, Merigan TC. Diagnosis of cytomegalovirus pneumonia in compromised hosts. Am J Med. 1976;61:326.
117. Jacobson MA, Mills J. Cytomegalovirus infection. Clin Chest Med. 1988;9:443.
118. Ballard RA, Drew WL, Hufnagle KG. Acquired cytomegalovirus infection in preterm infants. Am J Dis Child. 1979;133:482.
119. Gilbert GL, Hayes K, Hudson IL, et al. Prevention of transfusion-acquired cytomegalovirus infection in infants by blood filtration to remove leucocytes. Lancet. 1989;1:1228.
120. de Graan-Hentzen YCE, Gratama JW, Mudde GC. Prevention of primary cytomegalovirus infection in patients with hematologic malignancies by intensive white cell depletion of blood products. Transfusion. 1989;29:757.

121. Reverberi R, Menini C. Clinical efficacy of five filters specific for leukocyte removal. Vox Sang. 1990;58:188.

122. Brand A. White cell depletion: why and how. In: Nance SJ, ed. Transfusion Medicine in the 1990s. Arlington, Va: American Association of Blood Banks; 1990.

123. Bowen R, Sayers M. The risk of transmitting cytomegalovirus infection by fresh frozen plasma. Transfusion. 1990;30:762.

124. Epstein MA, Achong BG, Barr YM. Virus particles in cultured lymphoblasts from Burkitt's lymphoma. Lancet. 1964;2:702.

125. Jones JF. A perspective of Epstein-Barr virus diseases. Adv Pediatr. 1989;36:307.

126. McMonigal K, Horwitz CA, Henle W, et al. Post-perfusion syndrome due to Epstein-Barr virus. Transfusion. 1983;23:331.

127. Sumaya CV. Epstein-Barr virus serologic testing: diagnostic indications and interpretations. Pediatr Infect Dis. 1986;5:337.

128. Walker RH, ed. Technical Manual. 10th ed. Arlington, Va: American Association of Blood Banks; 1990:85.

129. Kieff E, Liebowitz D. Epstein-Barr virus and its replication. In: Fields BN, Knipe DM, eds. Virology. 2nd ed. New York, NY: Raven Press; 1990:1889-1958.

130. Yao QY, Rickinson AB, Epstein MA. A reexamination of the Epstein-Barr virus carrier state in healthy seropositive individuals. Int J Cancer. 1985;35:35.

131. Niederman JC. Infectious mononucleosis. In: Hoeprich PD, Jordan MC, eds. Infectious Diseases. Philadelphia, Pa: JB Lippincott; 1989.

132. Purcell RH, Walsh JH, Holland PV, et al. Seroepidemiological studies of transfusion-associated hepatitis. J Infect Dis. 1971;123:406.

133. Carter JW, Edson RS, Kennedy CC. Infectious mononucleosis in the older patient. Mayo Clin Proc. 1978;53:146.

134. Turner AR, MacDonald RN, Cooper BA. Transmission of infectious mononucleosis by transfusion of pre-illness plasma. Ann Intern Med. 1972;77:751.

135. Gallo RC, Nerurka LS. Human retroviruses: their role in neoplasia and immunodeficiency. Ann N Y Acad Sci. 1989;567:82.

136. Saxton EH, Lee H, Swanson P, et al. Detection of human leukemia/lymphoma virus type 1 in a transfused recipient with chronic myelopathy. Neurology. 1989;39:841.

137. Bove JR, Sandler SG. HTLV-I and blood transfusion. Transfusion. 1988;28:93.

138. Kim JH, Durack DT. Manifestations of human T-lymphotrophic virus type 1 infection. Am J Med. 1988;84:919.

139. Poiesz BJ, Ruscetti FW, Gasdar AF, et al. Detection and isolation of type C retrovirus particles from fresh and cultured lymphocytes of a patient with cutaneous T-cell lymphoma. Proc Natl Acad Sci. 1980;77:7415.

140. Kaplan JE, Khabbaz RF. HTLV-I: newest addition to blood donor screening. Am Fam Physician. 1989;40:189.

141. Rosenblatt JD, Chen ISY, Wachsman W. Infection with HTLV-I and HTLB-II: evolving concepts. Semin Hematol. 1988;25:230.

142. Hanada S, Uematsu T, Iwahashi M, et al. Prevalence of human T-cell leukemia virus type 1 infection in patients with hematologic and nonhematologic diseases in adult T-cell leukemia: endemic areas of Japan. Cancer. 1989;64:1290.

143. Shibasaki H, Endo C, Kuroda Y, et al. Clinical picture of HTLV-I associated myelopathy. J Neurol Sci. 1988;87:15.

144. Kawai H, Nishida Y, Takagi M, et al. HTLV-I associated myelopathy with adult T-cell leukemia. Neurology. 1989;39:1129.

145. Manns A, Blattner WA. The epidemiology of human T-cell lymphotrophic virus, type I and type II: etiologic role in human disease. Transfusion. 1991;31:67.

146. Shih JWK, Falchek LM, Canavaggio M, et al. Transfusion-transmitted HTLV-I/II infection in patients undergoing open heart surgery. Blood. 1990;75:546.

147. Canavaggio M, Leckie G, Allain JP, et al. The prevalance of antibody to HTLV-I/II in United States plasma donors, and in United States and French hemophiliacs. Transfusion. 1990;30:780.

148. Gottlieb MS, Schroff R, Schanker HM, et al. *Pneumocystis carinii* pneumonia and mucosal candidiasis in previously healthy homosexual men. N Engl J Med. 1981;305:1425.

149. Masur H, Michelis MA, Green JB, et al. An outbreak of community-acquired *Pneumocystis carinii* pneumonia. N Engl J Med. 1981;305:1431.

150. Siegal FP, Lopez C, Hammer G, et al. Severe acquired immunodeficiency in male homosexuals, manifested by chronic perianal ulcerative herpes simplex lesions. N Engl J Med. 1981;305:1439.

151. Safai B. Kaposi's sarcoma: a review of the classical and epidemic forms. Ann N Y Acad Sci. 1984;437:373.

152. Centers for Disease Control. Acquired immunodeficiency syndrome (AIDS) update: United States. MMWR. 1983;32:309.

153. Davis KC, Horsburgh CR, Hasiba U, et al. Acquired immunodeficiency syndrome in a patient with hemophilia. Ann Intern Med. 1983;3:284.

154. Evatt BL, Ramsey RB, Lawrence DN, et al. The acquired immunodeficiency syndrome in a patient with hemophilia. Ann Intern Med. 1984;100:499.

155. American Association of Blood Banks. Joint statement on acquired immune deficiency syndrome (AIDS) related to transfusion. Transfusion. 1983;23:87.

156. Simon TL, Bankhurst AD. A pilot study of surrogate tests to prevent transmission of acquired immune deficiency syndrome by transfusion. Transfusion. 1984;24:373.

157. Pindyck J, Waldman A, Zang E, et al. Measures to decrease the risk of acquired immunodeficiency syndrome transmission by blood transfusion. Transfusion. 1985;25:3.

158. Pindyck J. Transfusion-associated HIV infection. AIDS. 1988;2:239.

159. Barre-Sinoussi F, Chermann JC, Rey F, et al. Isolation of a T-lymphotropic retrovirus from a patient at risk for acquired immune deficiency syndrome (AIDS). Science. 1983;220:868.

160. Gallo RC, Salahuddin SZ, Popovic M, et al. Frequent detection and isolation of cytopathic retroviruses (HTLV-III) from patients with AIDS and at risk for AIDS. Science. 1984;244:500.

161. Melbye M, Froebel KS, Madhok R, et al. HTLV-III seropositivity in European haemophiliacs exposed to factor VIII concentrate imported from the USA. Lancet. 1984;1:1444.

162. Cumming PD, Wallace EL, Schorr JB, Dodd RY. Exposure of patients to human immunodeficiency virus through the transfusion of blood components that test antibody negative. N Engl J Med. 1989;321:941.

163. Menitov JE. Current risk of transfusion-associated human immunodeficiency virus infection. Arch Pathol Lab Med. 1990;114:330.

164. Levy JA. Human immunodeficiency viruses and the pathogenesis of AIDS. JAMA. 1989;261:2997.

165. Smith RD. Pathobiology of HIV infection. Arch Pathol Lab Med. 1990;114:235.

166. Greene WC. The molecular biology of human immunodeficiency virus type 1 infection. N Engl J Med. 1991;324:308.

167. Popovic M, Sarngadharan MG, Read E, Gallo RC. Detection, isolation, and continuous production of cytopathic retroviruses (HTLV-III) from patients with AIDS and pre-AIDS. Science. 1984;224:497.

168. Salahuddin SZ, Groopman JE, Markham PD, et al. HTLV-III in symptom free seronegative persons. Lancet. 1984;1:1418.

169. Horsburgh CR, Ou CY, Jason J, et al. Duration of human immunodeficiency virus infection before detection of antibody. Lancet. 1989;1:637.

170. Imagawa DT, Lee MH, Wolinsky SM, et al. Human immunodeficiency virus, type 1 infection in homosexual men who remain seronegative for prolonged periods. N Engl J Med. 1989;320:1458.

171. Ou WY, Kwok S, Mitchell SW, et al. DNA amplification for direct detection of HIV-l in DNA of peripheral blood mononuclear cells. Science. 1988;239:295.

172. Perrin LH, Yerly S, Adami N, et al. Human immunodeficiency virus DNA amplification and serology in blood donors. Blood. 1990;76:641.

173. Allain JP, Laurian Y, Paul DA, et al. Serological markers in early stages of human immunodeficiency virus infection in haemophiliacs. Lancet. 1986;2:1233.

174. Husson RN, Comeau AM, Hoff R. Diagnosis of human immunodeficiency virus infection in infants and children. Pediatrics. 1990;86:1.

175. Valdiserri RO, Taylor RN, Hearn TL, et al. Centers for Disease Control perspective on quality assurance for human immunodeficiency virus type 1 antibody testing. Arch Pathol Lab Med. 1990;114:263.

176. Dock NL, Lamberson HV, O'Brien TA, et al. Evaluation of atypical human immunodeficiency virus immunoblot reactivity in blood donors. Transfusion. 1988;28:412.

177. Fauci AS. The human immunodeficiency virus: infectivity and mechanisms of pathogenesis. Science. 1988;239:617.

178. Seligmann M, Pinching AJ, Rosen FS, et al. Immunology of human immunodeficiency virus and the acquired immunodeficiency syndrome. Ann Intern Med. 1987;107:234.

179. Centers for Disease Control. Revision of the CDC surveillance case definition for acquired immunodeficiency syndrome. MMWR. 1987;36(suppl 1):3.

180. Centers for Disease Control. Classification system for human immunodeficiency virus (HIV) infection in children under 13 years of age. MMWR. 1987;36:225.

181. Kessler HA, Blaauw B, Spear J, et al. Diagnosis of human immunodeficiency virus infection in seronegative homosexuals presenting with an acute viral syndrome. JAMA. 1987;258:1196.

182. Murray JF, Garay SM, Hopewell PC, et al. Pulmonary complications of the acquired immunodeficiency syndrome: an update. Am Rev Respir Dis. 1987;135:504.

183. White DA, Matthay RA. Noninfectious pulmonary complications of infection with the human immunodeficiency virus. Am Rev Respir Dis. 1989;140:1763.

184. Hiddemann W. What's new in malignant tumors in acquired immunodeficiency disorders? Pathol Res Pract. 1989;185:930.

185. Gabuzda DH, Hirsch MS. Neurologic manifestations of infection with human immunodeficiency virus. Ann Intern Med. 1987;107:383.

186. McArthur JC. Neurologic manifestations of AIDS. Medicine. 1987;66:407.

187. Price RW, Brew B, Sidtis J, et al. The brain in AIDS: central nervous system HIV-l infection and AIDS dementia complex. Science. 1988;239:586.

188. Gazzard BG. HIV disease and the gastroenterologist. Gut. 1988;29:1497.

189. Zon LI, Arkin C, Groopman JE. Haematologic manifestations of the human immune deficiency virus (HIV). Br J Haematol. 1987;66:251.

190. Perkocha LA, Rodgers GM. Hematologic aspects of human immunodeficiency virus infection. Am J Hematol. 1988;29:94.

191. Kaye BR. Rheumatologic manifestations of infection with human immunodeficiency virus (HIV). Ann Intern Med. 1989;111:158.

192. Coplan NL, Bruno MS. Acquired immunodeficiency syndrome and heart disease. Am Heart J. 1989;117:1175.

193. Humphreys MH, Schoenfeld PY. Renal complications in patients with the acquired immune deficiency syndrome. Am J Nephrol. 1987;7:1.

194. Warner LC, Fisher BK. Cutaneous manifestations of the acquired immunodeficiency syndrome. Int J Dermatol. 1986;25:337.

195. Landsman SH. Human immunodeficiency virus infection in women: an overview. Semin Perinatol. 1989;13:2.
196. Dinsmoor MJ. HIV infection and pregnancy. Med Clin North Am. 1989;73:701.
197. Falloon J, Eddy J, Wiener L, Pizzo PA. Human immunodeficiency virus infection in children. J Pediatr. 1989;114:1.
198. Katz BZ. Natural history and clinical management of the infant born to a mother infected with human immunodeficiency virus. Semin Perinatol. 1989;13:27.
199. Scutchfield FD, Benenson AS. AIDS update. Postgrad Med. 1989;84:289.
200. Peterman TA, Jaffee HW, Feorino PM, et al. Transfusion-associated acquired immunodeficiency syndrome in the United States. JAMA. 1985;254:2913.
201. Eyster ME, Goedert JJ, Sarngadharan MH, et al. Development and early natural history of HTLV antibodies in persons with hemophilia. JAMA. 1985;253:2219.
202. Peterman TA, Stoneburner RL, Allen JR, et al. Risk of human immunodeficiency virus transmission from heterosexual adults with transfusion-associated infections. JAMA. 1988;259:55.
203. Ranki A, Krohn M, Allain JP, et al. Long latency precedes overt seroconversion virus infection. Lancet. 1987;2:589.
204. Groopman JE, Caiazzo T, Thomas MA, et al. Lack of evidence of prolonged human immunodeficiency virus infection before antibody seroconversion. Blood. 1988;71:1752.
205. Ward JW, Deppe DA, Samson S, et al. Risk of human immunodeficiency virus infection from blood donors who later developed AIDS. Ann Intern Med. 1987;106:61.
206. Saulsbury FT, Wykoff RF, Boyle RJ. Transfusion-acquired human immunodeficiency virus infection in twelve neonates: epidemiologic, clinical and immunologic features. Pediatr Infect Dis J. 1987;6:544.
207. Perkins HA, Samson S, Garner J, et al. Risk of AIDS for recipients of blood components from donors who subsequently developed AIDS. Blood. 1987;70:1604.
208. Pruce GF, Lusher JM, Brownstein AP, et al. The use of purified clotting factor concentrates in hemophilia. JAMA. 1989;261:3434.
209. Borden CW, Hall WH. Fatal transfusion reactions from massive bacterial contamination of blood. N Engl J Med. 1951;245:760.
210. Myhre BA. Fatalities from blood transfusion. JAMA. 1980;244:1333.
211. Myhre BA. Bacterial contamination is still a hazard of blood transfusion. Arch Pathol Lab Med. 1985;109:982.
212. Pittman M. A study of bacteria implicated in transfusion reactions and bacteria isolated from blood products. J Lab Clin Med. 1953;42:273.
213. Zimmerman JJ, Dietrich KA. Current perspectives on septic shock. Pediatr Clin North Am. 1987;34:131.
214. Kreger BE, Craven DE, Carling PC, McCabe WR. Gram-negative bacteremia. Am J Med. 1980;68:332.
215. Houston MC, Thompson L, Robertson D. Shock, diagnosis and management. Arch Intern Med. 1984;149:1433.
216. Braude AI, Sanford JP, Bartlett JE, Mallery OT. Effects and clinical significance of bacterial contaminants in transfused blood. J Lab Clin Med. 1952;39:902.
217. Wood EE. Brucellosis as a hazard of blood transfusion. Br Med J. 1955;1:27.
218. Bjune G, Ruud TE, Eng J. Bacterial shock due to transfusion with *Yersinia enterocolitica*-infected blood. Scand J Infect Dis. 1984;16:411.
219. Ness PM, Perkins HA. Transient bacteremia after dental procedures and other minor manipulations. Transfusion. 1980;20:82.
220. Brown SE, White SE. *Yersinia enterocolitica* and transfusion-induced septicemia. Anesth Analg. 1988;67:415.

221. Walker RH, ed. Technical Manual. 10th ed. Arlington, Va: American Association of Blood Banks; 1990:118.

222. Myhre BA, Walker LJ, White ML. Bacteriocidal properties of platelet concentrates. Transfusion. 1974;14:116.

223. Chambers RW, Foley HT, Schmidt PJ. Transmission of syphilis by fresh blood components. Transfusion. 1969;9:32.

224. De Schryver A, Meheus A. Syphilis and blood transfusion. Transfusion. 1990;30:844.

225. Holmes KK, Lukehart SA. Syphilis. In: Braunwald E, ed. Harrison's Principles of Internal Medicine. 11th ed. New York, NY: McGraw-Hill; 1987:639-649.

226. Ravitch MM, Chambers JW. Spirochaetal survival in frozen plasma. Bull Johns Hopkins Hosp. 1942;71:299.

227. Turner TB, Diseker TH. Duration of infectivity of *Treponema pallidum* in citrated blood stored under conditions obtaining in the blood banks. Bull Johns Hopkins Hosp. 1941;68:269.

228. Long EG. Malaria. In: Balows A, Hausler WJ, Lennette EH, eds. Laboratory Diagnosis of Infectious Diseases. New York, NY: Springer-Verlag; 1988:911-928.

229. Dover AS, Schultz MG. Transfusion-induced malaria. Transfusion. 1971;11:353.

230. Walker RH, ed. Technical Manual. 10th ed. Arlington, Va: American Association of Blood Banks; 1990:6.

231. Cambell CC. Malaria. In: Hoeprich PD, Jordan MC, eds. Infectious Diseases. 4th ed. Philadelphia, Pa: JB Lippincott; 1989:1327-1337.

232. Plorde JJ, White NJ. Malaria. In: Braunwald E, ed. Harrison's Principles of Internal Medicine. 11th ed. New York, NY: McGraw-Hill; 1987:778-784.

233. Bruce-Chwatt LJ. Blood transfusion and tropical disease. Trop Dis Bull. 1972;69:825.

234. Thapa BR, Bhakoo ON. Neonatal malaria: a clinical study of congenital and transfusional malaria. J Trop Pediatr. 1987;33:266.

235. Imes GD, Neafie RC. Babesiosis. In: Binford CH, Connor DH, eds. Pathology of Tropical and Extraordinary Diseases. Washington, DC: Armed Forces Institute of Pathology; 1:1976.

236. Spielman A. Human babesiosis on Nantucket Island: transmission by nymphal Ixodes ticks. Am J Trop Med Hygiene. 1976;25:784.

237. Ruebush TK, Juranek DD, Chisholm ES, et al. Human babesiosis on Nantucket Island. N Engl J Med. 1977;297:825.

238. Ruebush TK, Cassaday PB, Marsh HJ, et al. Human babesiosis on Nantucket Island. Ann Intern Med. 1977;86:6.

239. Rosner F, Zarrabi MH, Benach JL, Habicht GS. Babesiosis in splenectomized adults. Am J Med. 1984;76:696.

240. Jacoby GA, Hunt JV, Kosinski, et al. Treatment of transfusion-transmitted babesiosis by exchange transfusion. N Engl J Med. 1986;303:1098.

241. Wittner M, Rowin KS, Tanowitz HB, et al. Successful chemotherapy of transfusion babesiosis. Ann Intern Med. 1982;96:601.

242. Marcus LC, Vaiigorsky JM, Fanning WL, et al. A case report of transfusion-induced babesiosis. JAMA. 1982;248:465.

243. Grabowski EF, Giardina PJV, Goldberg D, et al. Babesiosis transmitted by a transfusion of frozen-thawed blood. Ann Intern Med. 1982;96:466.

244. Gatanby PA. Reduced CD4+ T cells and candidiasis in absence of HIV infection. Lancet. 1988;2:1027-1028.

245. Hansen ER, Lisby S, Baadagaard O, et al. Abnormal function of CD4+ helper/inducer T lymphocytes in a patient with widespread human papillomavirus type 3–related infection. Arch Dermatol. 1990;126:1604-1608.

246. Pankhurst C, Peakman M. Reduced CD4+ T cells and severe oral candidiasis in absence of HIV infection. Lancet. 1989;1:672.

247. Unexplained CD4+ T-lymphocyte depletion in persons without evident HIV infection: United States. MMWR. 1992;41(30):541-544.

248. Testing for HIV in the public and private sectors: Oregon, 1988–1991. MMWR. 1992;41(32):581-591.

249. American Red Cross, Dodd RY. The risk of transfusion-transmitted infection. N Engl J Med. 1992;327(6):419-420.

250. Donahue JG, Muñoz A, Ness PM, et al. The declining risk of posttransfusion hepatitis C virus infection. N Engl J Med. 1992;327(6):369-373.

## CHAPTER 4

# IMMUNOLOGIC HAZARDS OF TRANSFUSION OF BLOOD COMPONENTS AND DERIVATIVES

## IMMUNOLOGIC REACTIONS INVOLVING RED BLOOD CELLS

Great attention has been focused in recent years on the alarming increase in infectious complications of transfusion, particularly with the advent of AIDS. We must not allow this preoccupation with such phenomena to obscure the occurrence of significant and occasionally life-threatening reactions of a noninfectious nature, which are also a reality today. The majority of such reactions are characterized by relatively mild immunologic manifestations of a more or less incidental nature, allergic or otherwise, and they frequently require only minor symptomatic attention from the physician. However, because of the inevitability of occasional human error, a certain minimum number of more severe reactions, particularly those involving red blood cells (RBCs), remain problematic in their association with a significant morbidity and mortality. Such reactions, which include immunologically mediated hemolytic occurrences both immediate and delayed, have been substantially reduced over the years. This has been accomplished by a host of factors: aggressive refinements in antibody screening; compatibility testing; accurate patient and specimen identification procedures; meticulous logistics; and rigorous quality assurance measures. Nonetheless, such reactions still take place with a frequency that amply justifies extreme vigilance in the handling of all transfusible blood products. Regardless of the impatience with which such vigilance is occasionally greeted by physicians, it should always be remembered that a mistake in transfusion cannot be undone, while its potential adverse consequences can only be reversed in many cases with great difficulty, and often at greater expense. The medical director of a blood bank or transfusion service, therefore, must remain staunchly vigilant and inflexible where patient safety is concerned.

Immunologically mediated transfusion reactions involving RBCs fall into 2 clinical categories: immediate and delayed. Clinical symptoms and signs occur during or shortly after the transfusion in the immediate category. Nothing untoward may be observed for several days in the delayed category. Generally, immediate reactions result from the transfusion of RBCs that are incompatible with a naturally occurring IgM antibody, such as anti-A or anti-B. Such reactions are frequently characterized by the rapid intravascular destruction of the antibody-labeled donor RBCs and by the variable but frequently severe systemic effects that result most often from the activation of multiple plasma systems (eg, complement pathway, coagulation cascade, plasma-kinin pathway, serotonin release, fibrinolytic pathway). The patient's final reaction from the complex interplay of all these factors may be composed, to some extent, of the disproportionate quantitative effects of 1 or more of them combined.

Immediate reactions relating to IgG antibodies tend to be clinically less severe for a variety of reasons, including, in many cases, less complement activation and therefore less intravascular hemolysis, and quantitatively less severe activation of the multiple pathways mentioned previously. However, as with all biologic phenomena, exceptions do occur.

Delayed transfusion reactions are usually the result of an incompatibility that exists between donor RBCs and recipient plasma and apparently are acquired after the transfusion rather than being present at the original time of compatibility testing. Most often this incompatibility results from the primary immunization of the recipient to the given blood group antigen on some previous occasion (eg, either transfusion or pregnancy). Such incompatibility does not become manifest as a detectable residual antibody level through ordinary compatibility testing techniques; nonetheless, it appears to result in the establishment of immunologic memory for that particular antigen. Subsequent transfusion with RBCs bearing that respective antigen may well lead to an anamnestic antibody response, with large amounts of IgG antibody (specific to the antigen in question) being generated over a few days. This will result in the labeling of the transfused cells, with their subsequent sequestration in the macrophage system, and possibly some degree of hemolysis.

## Factors Affecting the Immune Destruction of Red Blood Cells

The more important of these factors are summarized in Table 4-1.

### *Type and Subclass of Antibody*

The majority of severe, life-threatening reactions (with some exceptions) are caused by IgM antibodies directed against specific blood group antigens. These are most often the so-called naturally occurring "isoagglutinins," anti-A and anti-B, although examples of anti-$Le^a$, anti-Vel, anti-$Tj^a$ (-p+pl+$p^k$), and anti-H (also known as "Bombay" phenotype) predominantly manifest IgM antibodies that may give rise to severe hemolytic reactions. Other occasional examples include some anti-M and anti-N

| TABLE 4-1 | FACTORS INFLUENCING IMMUNE DESTRUCTION OF RED BLOOD CELLS |
|---|---|
| | 1. Type and subclass of antibody |
| | 2. Antibody concentration and avidity |
| | 3. Thermal range of antibody |
| | 4. Dosage of incompatible red blood cells |
| | 5. Degree of complement activation |
| | 6. Activation of the macrophage system |

antibodies, as well as IgM examples of antibodies to other blood group antigens, such as Rh or Kell. These usually occur in conjunction with high-titer IgG antibodies directed against the same antigens. Because of the pentameric structure of IgM antibodies, they are able to involve multiple antigenic sites simultaneously and are highly effective activators of the complement system (classic pathway). Thus, if they are active at physiologic temperatures (35°C to 38°C), they are frequently highly effective hemolysins. It appears overwhelmingly evident that the majority of life-threatening immediate hemolytic reactions involving intravascular hemolysis are caused predominantly by IgM anti-A or anti-B.

IgG antibodies are divided into 4 subclasses: IgG1, IgG2, IgG3, and IgG4. The significance of these antibodies in immune-mediated hemolytic reactions has recently been reviewed by Anstall. In the context of alloantibodies, 2 specific RBC antigens—those falling into subclasses IgG1 and IgG3—are highly significant for reduction in survival of antibody-labeled RBCs. This is true in terms of binding to specific antigenic sites on RBCs, binding and activating the classic complement pathway, and possessing Fc receptors that can bind to corresponding receptors on the surface of macrophages.[1,2] IgG3 antibodies are especially effective in this manner. To illustrate the high effectiveness of IgG3 antibodies as compared to other subclasses, note the observation that RBCs labeled with some 100 copies of IgG3 are phagocytized as readily and effectively as those labeled with 10,000 copies of IgG1.[2] Red blood cells labeled with IgG2 or IgG4 show virtually no reduction in survival time while in the circulation, because the geometry of these molecules, especially when correlating to flexibility at the hinge region, does not permit successful attachment to macrophage receptors.

Since IgG3 alloantibodies are highly efficient in promoting the clearance of antibody-labeled cells by the macrophage system, and since they also show the greater propensity for binding and activation of complement, immediate hemolytic reactions mediated by this subclass tend to be characterized by the rapid extracellular sequestration of compatible donor cells, with varying degrees of intravascular hemolysis that is occasionally severe.[3] IgG1 alloantibodies are much less efficient in promoting either extravascular sequestration or intravascular lysis. IgG1 is only of the order of 1% of that of IgG3. Intravascular destruction of RBCs, in the presence of complement and IgG1 antibodies, is also much less efficient.

Alloantibodies of other immunoglobulin classes (IgA, IgD, IgE) specifically directed against known RBC antigens do not appear to occur.[4] Some examples of IgA autoantibodies, however, have been documented in autoimmune hemolytic anemia.[5] Macrophage receptors do not seem to interact with the Fc portion of IgA.

***Antibody Concentration and Avidity***

A direct correlation exists between antibody concentration and the ability to sensitize RBCs. This relationship, however, may be considerably modified by the immunoglobulin class of the antibody concerned. A lower concentration of IgM is equal to or more effective than a high concentration of IgG1. Within any class of antibody, however, the more antigenic sites that are labeled on the RBC, the greater the likelihood of its sequestration or, in the case of complement-activating antibodies, its intravascular destruction.

The avidity of an antibody reflects the equilibrium constant of the particular antigen-antibody reaction concerned. Generally, the higher the avidity at a given concentration of antibody the more antigenic sites will be labeled. The subsequent history of such a labeled cell will depend largely on the immunoglobulin class of the labeling antibody. IgM antibodies at or near their thermal optimum generally bring about rapid complement activation and hemolysis; IgG3 and to a lesser extent IgG1 antibodies are more likely to result in extravascular cell destruction with lesser degrees of hemolysis.[2,6]

***Thermal Range of Antibody***

The thermal range of an antibody is clearly important in determining its ability to produce in vivo destruction of RBCs. Where the thermal optimum of an antibody is widely discrepant with normal body temperature, as in the case of many so-called "cold agglutinins," the antibody will have little or no clinical significance. In general, antibodies that are not demonstrably active at temperatures greater than 30°C are highly unlikely to be the cause of any clinical problem.[4,5,7] A case in point is anti-Le$^b$. Whereas anti-Le$^a$ may be of considerable clinical significance and, being IgM in character, may result in severe hemolytic reactions, anti-Le$^b$ is seldom associated with clinically significant activity. Most examples show little or no activity above 22°C. Le$^b$-positive RBCs labeled with Cr51 and administered in small doses to patients with anti-Le$^b$ whose thermal range does not exceed 22°C do not result in destruction of these cells; rather, they survive normally or near normally in the circulation.[8] By contrast, antibodies that demonstrate activity at temperatures less than

30°C should be regarded as highly likely to cause problems.[9,10] The closer the thermal optimum approaches the normal physiologic temperature, the greater the likelihood of the antibody's clinical significance. Also, it is important to distinguish between thermal optimum and thermal range. Whereas the thermal optimum of IgM anti-A may be below 30°C, its range is broad and activity at 37°C is still highly significant.

***Dosage of Incompatible RBCs***

The clinical severity of immediate hemolytic reactions, especially those mediated by IgM antibodies, is also proportional to the dosage of incompatible cells delivered into the antibody-containing milieu. It has been observed that small numbers of incompatible cells delivered into an antibody-containing environment are destroyed (or removed) quite rapidly—other factors being equal—whereas larger numbers of RBCs may appear to be removed at a somewhat slower pace. While the concentration of antibody is relatively small, RBC dosage may be important. Although small numbers of cells may be labeled and rapidly destroyed, much larger numbers of cells delivered to a relatively low concentration of antibody may create a dilutive effect, with the antibody molecules being more widely distributed over a much larger density of antigenic receptors. This process results in sparse labeling of individual cells, which is unlikely to cause immediate hemolysis but may induce a slower rate of removal from the circulation. Again, if the antibody is unlikely to effect the rapid and complete activation of the classic complement pathway, then the presence in the circulation of large numbers of antibody-labeled RBCs may soon exceed the capacity of the macrophage system to phagocytize all of them. For a time, this may result in the assistance of sensitized incompatible cells. These observations are important when interpreting Cr51 RBC survival curves. The small number of Cr51-labeled cells injected may be removed rapidly in the presence of antibody, whereas if much larger doses were given, a better survival rate might prevail. When markedly incompatible cells are delivered into a high concentration of antibody, however, as in severe ABO incompatibilities in which complement activation is a prominent feature, large numbers of cells may be quickly destroyed in the circulation. The result produced is one of significant hemoglobinemia, hemoglobinuria, and other visceral and systemic effects associated with intravascular RBC destruction. In this context, it should be observed that dosage of incompatible RBCs correlates roughly with morbidity: a fatal outcome in such a reaction is unusual with dosages of less than 200 mL. As with all biologic systems, however, exceptions do occur. Occasionally fatal reactions with much smaller volumes have been documented.

In the same context, it is pertinent to consider the number of antigenic receptors of the antigen corresponding to a given antibody. The ease and degree to which RBCs may become sensitized to a given antibody correlate closely with the number of specific antigenic receptors that correspond to that antibody per unit surface area of cell membrane. The number of antibody molecules of immunoglobulin classes that can be accommodated per unit surface area increases proportionate to the antigenic density. If the antibody in question is able to bind and activate complement efficiently, the likelihood of cell destruction increases. This is well illustrated by the observation that cells that are homozygous for a particular antigen frequently show significantly greater antibody binding and much more accelerated cell removal or destruction than those that are heterozygous for the same antigen. This "dosage effect" of zygosity is often striking. A cell that is heterozygous for a gene determining a particular antigen can be expected to express only 50% of the antigenic receptor sites that would be exhibited by a cell homozygous for the same gene. This dosage effect may be striking in blood group systems where even in homozygous individuals the total number of antigenic determinants is not very large. In such systems, if heterozygous cells are used in RBC screening panels, weak antibodies might easily be missed. It is important to ascertain that the screening cells used for detection of such antibodies are homozygous for the antigen in question. Similarly, the distribution of such antigenic receptors over the surface of the cell membrane may be important, in addition to the total number present. For example, in some antigens the distribution cannot be assumed to be uniform, and in some cases antigenic receptors appear to exhibit a degree of mobility within the cell membrane, forming clusters of greater density in some areas with a sparser distribution elsewhere. This is of particular importance when dealing with antigens to which the corresponding antibodies are IgG. Complement will only be activated where IgG molecules can bind to 2 adjacent receptor sites.[11] The full implications of such variable antigenic density have yet to be determined for any blood group system.[2]

### *Degree of Complement Activation*

A number of distinct but correlated factors influence the degree to which the classic complement pathway is activated: immunoglobulin class or IgG subclass; thermal range and temperature optimum of the antibody concerned; antigenic density and distribution; and the degree of sensitization of the RBC. These factors weigh also in determining the degree to which this activation proceeds in a given situation.

Figure 4-1 illustrates the classic pathway in a somewhat simplified summary form. The appropriate binding of a complement-activating antibody to its antigenic receptor on the RBC membrane may initiate the classic pathway through the binding of the first component of complement, C1, resulting in the activation of the previously inert C1 to an enzymatically active form: C1s. This in turn interacts with 2 other components of the complement system, C4 and C2, generating 2 immediate products: C4b and the complex C4b2a. C4b becomes attached to the cell membrane as a single entity, while C4b2a functions enzymatically as a C3 convertase.

**FIGURE 4-1** Activation of the classic complement pathway bringing about immune destruction of RBCs in hemolytic transfusion reactions.

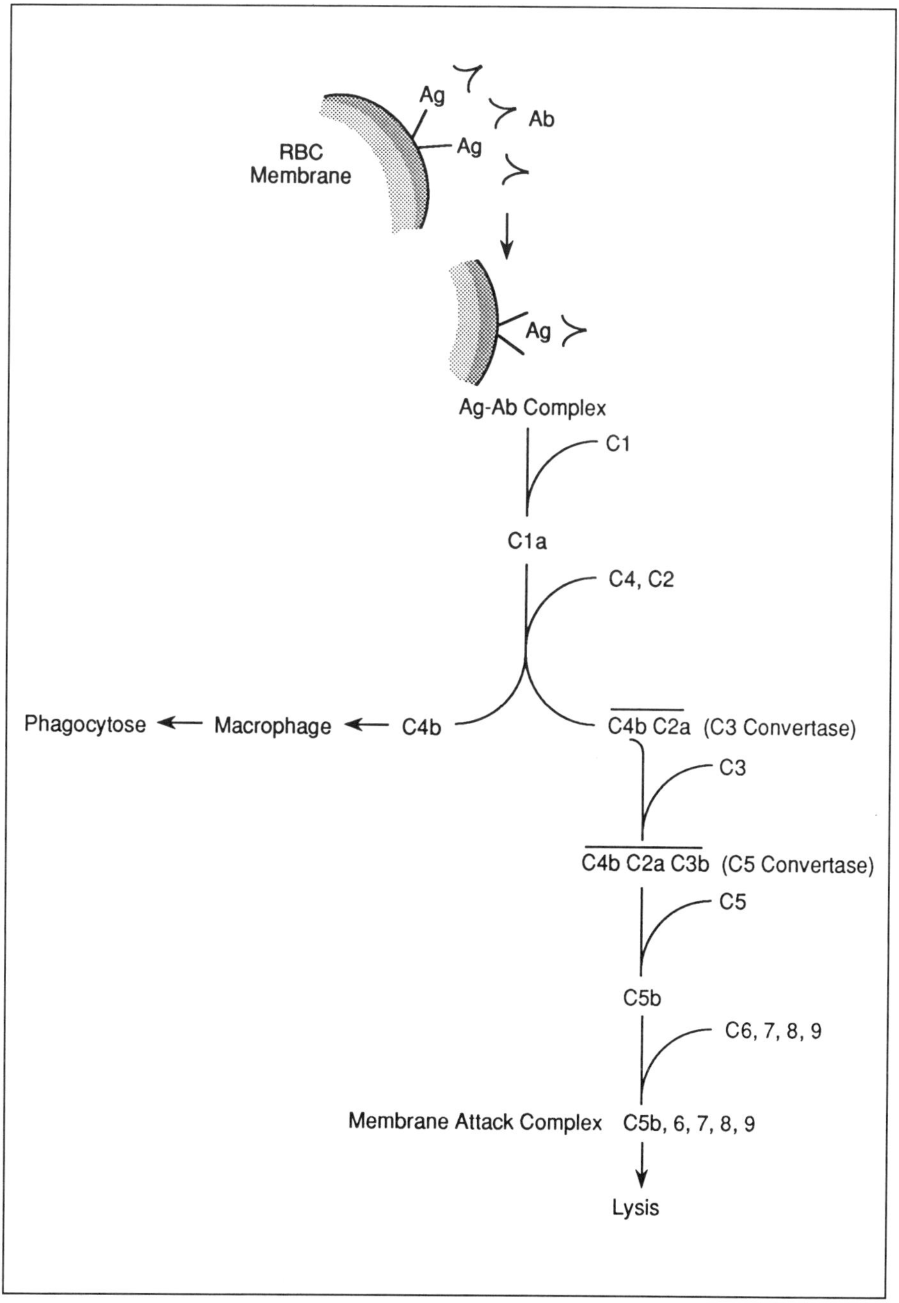

The fate of the RBC sensitized by antibody and possessing some degree of complement activation depends largely on the degree to which the activation of the classic pathway continues. If activation does not proceed significantly beyond the C4b stage, then sequestration of the antibody-sensitized and C4b-coated cells can be expected to follow, resulting in reduction of the circulating life span. Conversely, generation of efficient C3 convertase will produce the enzymatically active complex C5 convertase (C4bC2aC3b), which will lead to the conversion of C5 to C5b. The subsequent incorporation of C6, C7, C8, and C9 leads to the generation of the "membrane attack complex" (Figure 4-1). The complement components, C6 and C7, are bound by C5b in a nonenzymatic step. The further incorporation of components C8 and C9 may then occur but may be competitively inhibited by lipoprotein, antithrombin III, or protein.[5] If the binding of C8 and C9 to the C5bC6C7 complex proceeds to a significant degree, however, the resulting membrane attack complex will permit the highly lyophilic terminal of this complex to penetrate the bimolecular lipid core of the membrane, causing local destabilization and disruption. This process repeated hundreds of times over the surface of the cell membrane will have an effect reminiscent of that of a shotgun blast. It will produce a constellation of focal penetrations and dislocations of the membrane with its consequent collapse and perforation. In the case of the circulating RBCs, this is intravascular hemolysis.[12] The essential difference between intravascular and extravascular phagocytosis of antibody and/or complement-labeled RBCs depends primarily on the degree of activation of the classic pathway. Where this does not proceed significantly beyond the formation of C4b, the RBC will suffer extravascular phagocytosis. When the activation proceeds to the generation of the membrane attack complex, as in IgM-mediated reactions, rapid intravascular destruction is the rule.

The sensitivity of RBCs has been observed to modulate somewhat with varying levels of complement system activation. For example, the cells of patients with paroxysmal nocturnal hemoglobinuria (PNH) are exquisitely sensitive to almost any degree of complement activation, and thus require transfusion. The use of frozen, deglycerolized, saline-suspended RBCs is generally recommended to avoid the transfusion of plasma, which would introduce complement components and the inherent possibility of complications. Even a minor immunologic event (such as an allergic reaction) could lead to a limited degree of complement deactivation, an occurrence sufficient to precipitate hemolysis of these complement-sensitive, structurally abnormal cells. Again, under such circumstances, the transfusion of group O plasma into a group A recipient might lead to sufficient complement activation to create some degree of hemolysis. Disagreement still prevails concerning the need for using washed or deglycerolized frozen RBCs. Where no disparity exists between ABO group types, however, many physicians would prefer to avoid transfusion of heterologous plasma, considering this a desirable alternative.[13,14]

### *Activation of the Macrophage (RE) System*

There appears to be significant variability in the ease with which macrophages recognize antibody and/or complement-labeled RBCs. This process of recognition seems to differ between persons and to some extent within the same person.[15,16] Persons who show the HLA haplotype HLAB8/DRw exhibit varying degrees of Fc receptor dysfunction.[17] Those who have certain autoimmune diseases characterized by periodic circulation of immune complexes (eg, systemic lupus erythematosus and rheumatoid arthritis and its variants) may exhibit similar disturbances in macrophage function. This condition affects their ability to phagocytize antibody or complement-labeled RBCs.[18,19] Steroids appear to be capable of triggering suppression of Fc receptor function to some extent.[17] These factors, in addition to those previously discussed, appear to influence the rate at which antibody and/or complement-labeled cells are cleared from the circulation.

## Immediate Hemolytic Reaction

### *Pathogenesis*

Most immediate hemolytic reactions are initiated by the interaction of IgM antibodies, with their corresponding antigenic receptors on transfused incompatible donor cells, followed by the rapid activation of the classic complement pathway, which results in a sometimes considerable degree of intravascular lysis. The majority of these reactions are due to ABO incompatibilities and therefore to human error. Occasionally, however, other blood group system antibodies are involved, some IgM and others IgG, most particularly of subclasses 3 or 1. Table 4-2 summarizes the various antibodies that are most usually implicated in reactions of this kind. Characteristically, most efficient, immediate RBC destruction is likely to result from IgM antibodies with a broad-enough thermal range to be active at 37°C. A significant spectrum of severity may also occur from avid, complement-binding IgG antibodies. These may include examples of IgG anti-A and anti-B, especially in group O persons. The various antibodies involved in immediate reactions have been conveniently reviewed by Greenwalt[20] and Mollison.[21] "Minor-side" incompatibility (between transfused plasma and recipient RBCs) has been documented, even though it is of lower incidence because of transfused antibody dilution. This condition usually results from transfusion of large amounts of group O whole blood or plasma to A, AB, or B recipients. Most examples are caused by plasmas containing potent anti-A1 activity, with actual immediate hemolysis occurring in some 1% of subjects, and delayed hemolysis occurring more extensively.[22] Reactions resulting from this "passive transfer" of anti-A or anti-B antibody have been reported sporadically where the use of a wide variety of blood components and derivatives is present. This is especially true where large quantities have been used, including whole blood,[23,24] RBC concentrates,[25] platelet concentrates,[26-28] plasma,[29-34] factor VIII,[35-37] and human immunoglobulin operations.[36,37] When group O subjects are used as transplantation donors, either for bone marrow or for solid organs, a transfer of immunocompetent B cells together with the graft can result in the production of potent antibodies. These may include anti-A1, which when directed against the recipient's native RBCs results in hemolysis.[38-43]

Union of a complement-activating antibody with its corresponding antigen on the surface of the RBC in vivo generates a number of normally inert precursors, which in turn may lead to the progressive activation of complement, coagulation, kinin, and fibrinolytic systems. Complete activation of the classic pathway leads to intravascular hemolysis, which liberates RBC contents into the surrounding medium. In most major immediate hemolytic reactions, some 50% to 90% of the incompatible cells are likely to undergo rapid lysis. Thus, large amounts of hemoglobin may be rapidly liberated, depending on the dosage of cells administered. This hemoglobin, now free in plasma, may undergo fairly rapid dissociation into dimeric components, and the heme portion is quickly oxidized to methemoglobin. Hemoglobin also undergoes partial separation of the heme component, which is conserved. The globin entity, together with varying amounts of intact hemoglobin, become bound to haptoglobin in

**TABLE 4-2 | PRINCIPAL ANTIBODIES INVOLVED IN IMMEDIATE-TYPE HEMOLYTIC TRANSFUSION REACTIONS**

| Antibody | Usual Ig Class | Mostly Intravascular Hemolysis | Mostly Extravascular RBC Destruction |
|---|---|---|---|
| Anti-A,B,H | IgM (Some IgG in group O) | Yes | No |
| Anti-$Le^a$ | IgM | Yes | No |
| Some Anti $P_1$, M, N, S, Vel | IgM or IgG | Variable | Variable |
| Anti-D ($Rh_o$) | IgG III, IgG I | No | Yes |
| Other Rh Abs | IgG III, IgG I | No | Yes |
| Anti-$Fy^a$, $By^b$, Ka | IgG III, IgG I | No | Yes |
| Anti-$Jk^a$, $Jk^b$ | IgG III, IgG I | No | Yes |
| High-titer, low-avidity Abs (HTLA) | IgG | Usually no | Some |

plasma. Methemoglobin and the oxidized product of separated hememetheme are selectively bound by hemopexin. Any excess of heme or metheme, over that removed by 20 hemopexin, is bound to serum albumin, which then forms methalbumin. The carrier proteins, haptoglobin and hemopexin, provide a mechanism for the selective and sequential removal of hemoglobin and its various degradation products. The rapid liberation of hemoglobin from even relatively small numbers of RBCs and the more or less immediate binding of intact hemoglobin and hemoglobin dimers by haptoglobin result in the rapid saturation of haptoglobin binding capacity. Thus, even relatively small amounts of hemolysis create a rapid reduction in haptoglobin levels. At the same time, if amounts of hemoglobin separated are not such as to leave an excess in plasma unbound to haptoglobin, which could then readily undergo oxidation to free methemoglobin and metheme, then hemopexin levels could be relatively normal, whereas haptoglobin levels could be greatly reduced. In this instance, haptoglobin/hemoglobin complexes are removed by the macrophage system, the iron of hemoglobin is conserved, and the globin moiety undergoes degradation.

When the binding capacity of the carrier proteins is exceeded, the excess of hemoglobin is filtered at the glomerulus and begins to appear in the urine. This will occur at levels in excess of the initial binding capacity of haptoglobin, and commonly at plasma hemoglobin levels of 150 mg/dL or greater. Hemoglobin dimers readily pass the glomerular filter at approximately 5% of the inulin clearance rate.[44] About 30% of this hemoglobin dimer is reabsorbed in the proximal convoluted tubule, while a portion of the iron is being separated and conserved in the form of ferritin. Some, however is lost as frank hemoglobin, and some appears in the urine as ferritin/hemosiderin granules, which can be shown to stain positively with Prussian blue. It then follows that intravascular destruction of small amounts of RBCs will not ordinarily result in hemoglobinuria, since the amount of hemoglobulin liberated can generally be accommodated by plasma haptoglobin and by hepatic metabolism of heme.

In this latter context, free plasma hemoglobin may be absorbed directly by the liver. If this occurs, the heme is broken down, with the iron being conserved and the porphyrin moiety being converted to bilirubin. In significant hemolytic reactions the amount of heme presented to the liver for metabolism may generate sufficient bilirubin to temporarily exceed the conjugating capacity of the hepatocyte, so that the principal increase in plasma bilirubin observed in such circumstances is that of unconjugated ("indirectly reacting") bilirubin.

It has been known for some years that complement-binding and complement-activating immune complexes appear to bring about the direct activation of the precursors of other systems capable of being mobilized in plasma. Through this mechanism, the intrinsic coagulation cascade can be set in motion leading ultimately to the generation of fibrin (Figure 4-2). Simultaneously, liberation of thromboplastic intracellular components from lysed RBCs will reinforce this effect by simultaneously activating the extrinsic coagulation pathway. The probable result of these actions is the production of varying degrees of disseminated intravascular coagulation (DIC) characterized by the rapid consumption of soluble procoagulants (factors V, VIII, prothrombin, fibrinogen, together with platelets). Fibrin may be deposited on the surface of larger blood vessels, while fibrin thrombi (plugs) may be widely deposited in the lumina of small blood vessels (eg, those of the renal glomerulus and of the peritubular capillary network), activating various levels of destruction and circulatory interruption. In the kidney, the clinical result of such a process will be expressed by the sum of all of these microcirculatory occlusions. If sufficient glomeruli are obstructed, the glomerular filtration rate (GFR) will fall in proportion. When the GFR is large, severe oliguria or complete anuria may result. Again, multiple plugging of peritubular capillaries may lead to a patchy ischemia of segments of the renal tubules, especially of the proximal convoluted tubules. This will lead to the infarction of varying lengths of epithelial cells, with islets of less compromised or even normal areas in between. It is uncommon in most cases for total necrosis of the tubular epithelium to occur because of the extensive anastomotic connections between the peritubular capillaries. Islands of normal or mildly hypoxic epithelial cells will survive occasionally as isolated colonies among areas of frank necrosis and sloughing. Sometimes, however, the vascular compromise is great enough to permit apparent total and irreversible destruction of tubular epithelium, resulting in so-called "bilateral cortical necrosis." We can thus postulate 2 basic renal lesions that may result from antibody-mediated acute intravascular hemolysis: glomerular obstruction with reduction of GFR and oliguria/anuria with varying degrees of acute tubular necrosis and compromise of the kidney's concentrating/diluting capability.[45-47] A further complication of DIC is hemorrhage, which can be life threatening.

Activation of the plasma-kinin system (Figure 4-3) may be a consequence of the concurrent activation of the intrinsic coagulation pathway and may lead to the rapid and the generally early generation of pharmacologically significant amounts of bradykinin. Activated Hageman factor (XIIa) may bring about activation of prekallikrein activator (PKA), which will in turn activate the inert precursor polypeptide, prekallikrein, to kallikrein. The enzymic removal of the terminal peptide from kininogen converts it into the pharmacologically active bradykinin. The name "polypeptide" was derived from its ability to bring about the slow, sustained contraction of guinea pig uterine smooth muscle. This system was once used as a bioassay method for measuring bradykinin in biologic fluids. However, the results of bradykinin activity vary with the location and the nature of the smooth muscle. In arteriolar smooth muscle,

**FIGURE 4-2** Activation of the intrinsic coagulation pathway by RBC membrane-bound immune complexes.

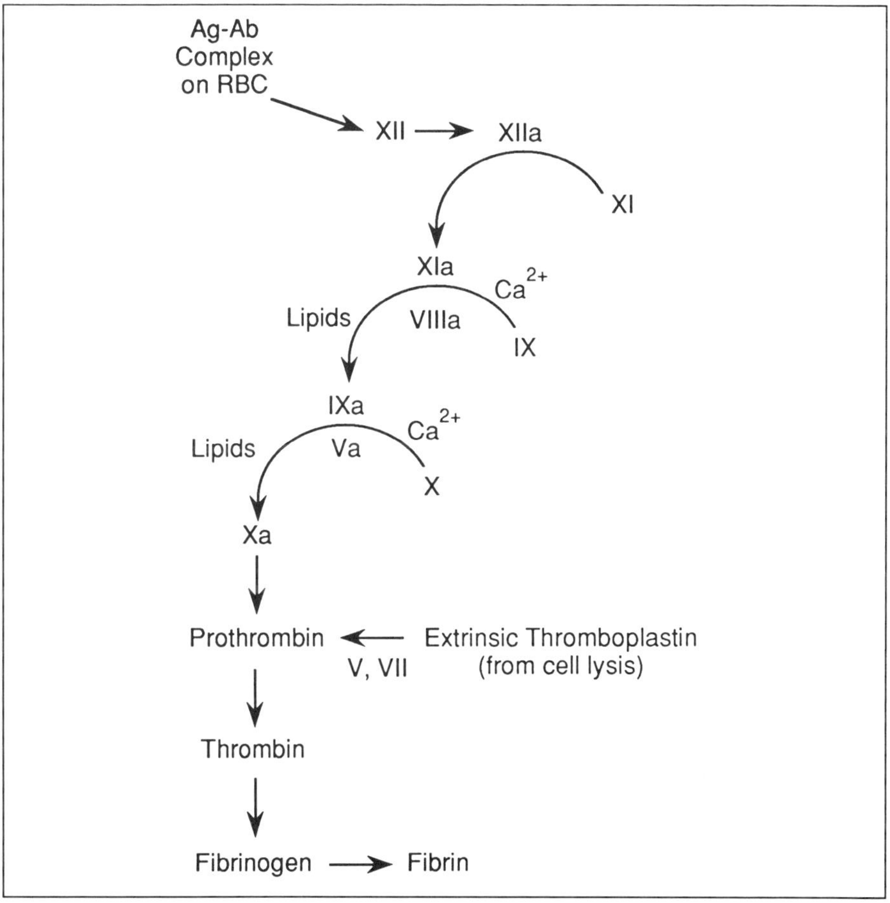


bradykinin is able to bring about a relaxation of the arteriolar sphincter with consequent shunting of blood from the arterial to the capillary/venous side, with a sometimes considerable reduction in mean arterial pressure. The patient may experience light-headedness, fainting, or even severe or life-threatening shock. The action of complement fragments (C3a, C5a, C567 complex) and a variety of effector cells, including mast cells, may produce other pharmacologic effects (eg, the release of various vasoactive compounds, including serotonin and histamine.

Variable amounts of catecholamines may be released from the adrenal medulla during the hemolytic reaction as a general response to stress. The overall systemic effects will depend on the amount released and the

**FIGURE 4-3** | Activation of the plasma-kinin system during the course of a hemolytic transfusion reaction.

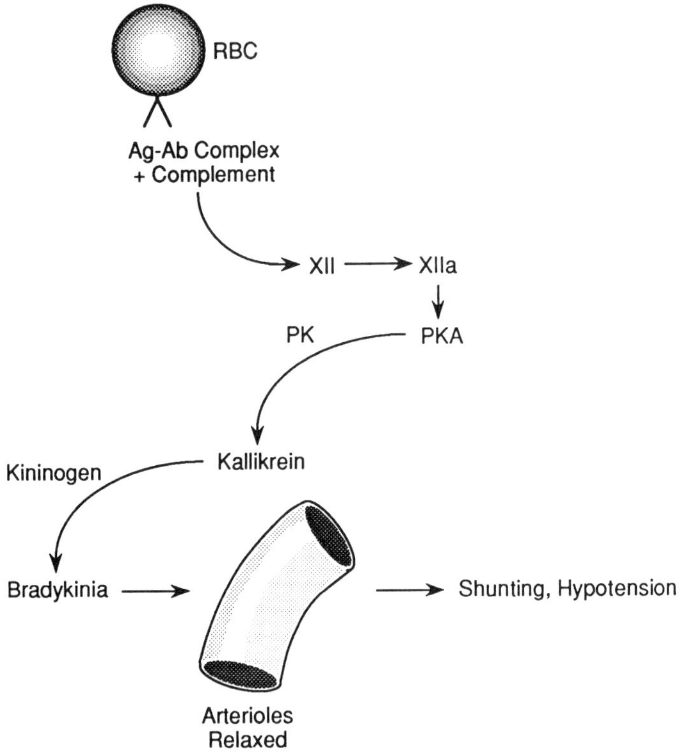


relative quantities of epinephrine and norepinephrine. Similarly, the amount of catecholamine released relative to the amount of bradykinin generated will largely determine the effect on blood pressure. Where these are pharmacologically balanced, little or no effect on blood pressure may be observed. In some cases where catecholamine production exceeds kinin generation theoretically, there may even be a transient rise in pressure.[1]

The importance of complement activation in the generation of many of these adverse biologic consequences should be emphasized. Blood group–specific antibodies that merely label RBCs but do not activate the classic complement pathway are not associated with severe side effects due to coagulation pathway and kinin system activation. Nonimmunologically mediated hemolysis is not complicated by these biochemical events. For such side effects to occur, activation of the complement pathway appears to be necessary beyond the incorporation of C3.

Varying degrees of activation of the fibrinolytic system with conversion of plasminogen to plasmin may also complicate major hemolytic reactions. Although this may militate against some of the effect of DIC by the removal of fibrin deposits, it may also complicate the situation further by digestion and destruction of soluble procoagulants, thereby leaving the blood incoagulable and increasing the potential for hemorrhage.

***Clinical Features***

Table 4-3 lists the principal symptoms and signs associated with immediate hemolytic reactions. For convenience, emphasis is placed on those that are characteristic of more mild reactions as contrasted with severe or life-threatening ones, but the differences are only of degree. In about 70% of cases where intravascular hemolysis occurs, fever often elevated by 2 or 3 degrees and accompanied by chills is present. Stimulation of the thermoregulatory center in the brain stem by pyrogenic products when liberated from hemolyzed RBCs may produce this result. Alternatively, fever may be a manifestation of a WBC-related reaction mediated by anti-HLA antibodies, which would indicate a different mechanism and a different prognosis.

Frequent clinical features observed are burning and itching along the course of the vein receiving the incompatible RBCs, together with deep-seated, throbbing pain in the lumbar region. These reactions are often, though not always, bilateral and symmetric. Their symptoms, though somewhat obscure, are believed to represent a response to bradykinin-mediated stimulation of pain receptors in veins or in the renal vasculature. Anxiousness, breathlessness, a feeling of impending doom, and tachycardia may result from catecholamine secretion as part of the general stress reaction often accompanying the reaction. The potential for changes in blood pressure has been previously discussed: hypotension is more often observed than hypertension. This is due to the disproportionate release in moderate or severe reactions of bradykinin and other vasoactive amines. In more serious cases, hypotension may be severe enough to result in shock, which may be life threatening. Widespread and uncontrollable capillary oozing in patients undergoing surgery may also cause DIC. This in turn will result in clinical hemorrhage and an extensive blood loss. Hemoglobinuria will be observed in many cases.

A few comments with respect to hemoglobinuria are pertinent. It was formally thought that the renal damage and functional disturbance frequently seen in immediate hemolytic reactions resulted primarily from the toxic effects of hemoglobin on renal tubular epithelium and in reduction or occlusion of renal tubular outflow due to the accumulation of hemoglobin microcrystals where the urine pH was less than 7.0. Numerous experimental observations over the years, however, have led to the conclusion that hemoglobin is not significantly toxic to tubular epithelium (unlike myoglobin) and that crystalline hemoglobin does not

| Table 4-3 | Principal Clinical Features of Hemolytic Transfusion Reactions |
|---|---|
| | Associated with Mild Reactions<br>Anxiety, fever, chills, flushing, low back pain, mild hypotension<br><br>Associated with Severe Reactions<br>All the above with dyspnea and precordial pain, hemoglobulinurea, shock, capillary bleeding, and oliguria/anuria |

produce mechanical obstruction of renal tubules. Hemoglobin, therefore, cannot be considered a significant contributor to the renal lesions of transfusion reactions.[48,49]

### *Laboratory Confirmation*

In a patient showing symptoms and signs suggestive of a major hemolytic reaction, prompt action must be taken to confirm the presence or absence of such a state so that precious time is not lost in instituting the appropriate management. Any untoward symptom or sign developing during the course of a blood transfusion should be a signal for its immediate interruption. While transfusion should be stopped, the intravenous line should be kept open by a slow infusion of normal saline. From the first signs it is obvious that a major incompatibility is present. One can tell at a glance that an inappropriate unit has been administered by checking the blood label and patient identification data. In other circumstances, no such incongruity may be apparent, and final diagnosis may depend on laboratory data.

Immediately stop the transfusion and keep the intravenous line open. The following samples should be drawn immediately from a vein other than the one into which the transfusion was given, and preferably from the opposite arm: 1) an anticoagulated sample (EDTA, purple-top tube); 2) a clotted specimen (red-top tube) for serologic screening and repeat of crossmatch; 3) a citrated sample (blue-top tube) for baseline coagulation parameters. These samples should be sent immediately to the laboratory for examination. The blood bag should also be promptly returned to the laboratory, and a specimen of the first voided urine after the event is also useful.

In the laboratory, the following procedures should be undertaken immediately. On receipt of the specimens, There should be no delay in performing the following tests:

1) A direct antiglobulin test (direct Coombs' test) should be performed on RBCs from the EDTA tube.
2) The EDTA tube is now centrifuged and the supernatant plasma immedi-

ately examined for free plasma hemoglobin. If the plasma is frankly red or pink, an absolute measurement of the hemoglobin level is of little value, since it is clear that frank hemolysis of significant degree is present. If the plasma is dubiously pink, a specimen may be sent for immediate determination of plasma hemoglobin. Free hemoglobin in plasma (ie, hemoglobin external to RBCs) becomes detectable by the human eye at concentrations of 25 mg/dL. If there is no suspicion of pink coloration, then only a very minor degree of hemolysis (if any) may be present. In our laboratory, the normal reference range for plasma-free hemoglobin is 0 to 7 mg/dL. In patients undergoing transfusion, values of up to 14 mg/dL are not uncommon and probably reflect free hemoglobin levels in the plasma of blood or RBC units stored under blood bank conditions.

3) Baseline coagulation parameters (eg, prothrombin time [PT], partial thromboplastin time [PTT], and presence of fibrin degradation products [FDPs]) should be determined to see if there is evidence of DIC. This discovery procedure will serve as a basis for comparison for possible future determinations. It is useful to examine a new blood smear from the patient for RBC morphology (presence of schistocytosis, microspherocytosis) and to form a rough estimate of platelet numbers.
4) The blood type of the patient and that of the unit in question should be redetermined and the unit recrossmatched using both pretransfusion and posttransfusion serum samples from the recipient.
5) A urine sample, if available, should be examined for the presence of hemoglobin (centrifuged) and the deposit examined for RBCs. When possible, a Prussian blue reaction is helpful to demonstrate the presence of blue-staining hemosiderin particles, particularly in association with cellular debris, where present. Distinguishing between hemoglobinuria and hematuria is often important, since the distinction may not be apparent on simple inspection. These conditions, under certain circumstances, may even coexist.

More sophisticated studies, including haptoglobin and hemopexin determinations, which will show marked decreases in the presence of significant hemolysis, and methemalbumin detection, may be of use primarily in examining patients with suspected lesser degrees of hemolysis. In the presence of a major immediate hemolytic reaction, such determinations are generally pointless.

Even though diagnosis may be certain before laboratory data are available, it may valuable from the clinical perspective to attain baseline electrolyte, urea nitrogen, and creatinine values to establish future comparisons for evaluation of renal function later.

### *Clinical Management and Prognosis*

Clinical management of an immediate hemolytic transfusion reaction is dictated by the pathogenesis of the syndrome and is aimed at the prevention or correction of those components of the syndrome that may become responsible for serious complications or death. As we have seen, the first critical step is to terminate the transfusion and thus to limit as much as possible the dosage of incompatible RBCs administered. Beyond this, therapy is aimed at the following: 1) control and reversal of hypotension or shock; 2) prevention or management of DIC and of clinical hemorrhage; 3) maintenance of renal function and an attempt to prevent serious renal complications.

Simple hypotension may be manageable merely by placing the patient in a prone position or by raising the foot of the bed, combined if necessary with intravenous infusion of normal saline. More severe degrees of hypotension or of overt shock may need vigorous treatment with pressor agents. Dopamine is the agent of choice, since it exhibits both alpha and beta adrenergic effects and will thus increase both peripheral resistance and cardiac output.[50-52] Dopamine is also believed to improve perfusion through the peritubular vascular network of the kidneys and thus to protect to some degree against ischemia. Selective vasospasm in this microcirculation may result from imbalances between various vasoactive materials liberated during the reaction, and may therefore produce ischemia.

Dopamine is given by intravenous infusion at a rate of 1 mg/kg of body weight per hour. This dosage is sufficient to maintain a systolic blood pressure of 100 mm Hg or higher, with careful monitoring of blood pressure, ECG, and cardiac output. Dopamine should not be used in hypovolemic patients, and any significant volume deficit must be promptly corrected before its use. A clinical indication for transfusion of blood or blood components may still exist. If so, these transfusions should not be withheld, but their compatibility must be established before they are used.

Determination of basic coagulation parameters (PT, PTT, FDPs) should be made at the earliest possible time. If these are shown to be marginal or abnormal, heparin therapy should be considered if no major clinical contraindication exists. Clearly there are many circumstances in which heparin therapy might be fraught with danger. Where these situations are not present, the early and judicious administration of heparin may prevent or abort the development of a florid DIC with its attendant risks of hemorrhage and of significant kidney damage. In this context, initial intravenous administration of heparin should be considered in doses of 40 IU (about 5000 IU for the average patient), followed by a similar dosage over the next 10 to 12 hours. The primary objective of this course of action is to prevent a progressive escalation of DIC and the development of a severe consumptive coagulopathy. Attendant consequences of the latter condition are possible hemorrhage and fibrin thrombus deposition, which is 1 of the principal determining factors of renal functional impairment, as observed in transfusion reactions. If a major DIC is already established, or if there are serious clinical contraindications to heparin, appropriate transfusion therapy using blood components (fresh frozen plasma, platelet concentrates, cryoprecipitate) should be administered as indicated. Under such circumstances, a transfusion physician should be called in consultation.

Protection of the kidney and maintenance of adequate renal function are also of critical importance in the management of immediate hemolytic reactions. It is also of major importance to obtain baseline parameters (electrolyte values, blood urea nitrogen, and creatinine concentration) and to monitor as accurately as possible the patient's fluid balance. The administration of certain diuretics may be valuable in these patients not, as formerly believed, to "flush the tubules and remove hemoglobin crystals." Rather, it is helpful to monitor the kidneys' ability to respond to the diuretic. This procedure aids the physician in evaluating the kidneys' functional status in order to maintain adequate urine output and to assist in maintaining adequate perfusion of the renal cortex. Evidence shows that diuretics such as furosemide (Lasix) and ethacrynic acid possess dilatory effects on the peritubular vascular network and may thus be of value in maintaining adequate perfusion and in reducing ischemic necrosis of tubular epithelial cells.[53-56] Furosemide can be intravenously administered in an initial dose of 20 mg, repeated as frequently as is necessary to maintain a urine output of not less than 100 mL/hr. This dosage should be maintained for at least 12 hours, by which time the immediate danger of acute renal failure is likely to be past. Careful attention must be paid to prevent insensible perspiration as well as urinary loss or any losses through vomiting or other sources.

Mannitol is an alternative diuretic whose mechanism's action is primarily osmotic rather than on the renal tubular epithelial cells. This drug may be administered as a 20% solution, up to a total dose of 100 g over a 24-hour period. Earlier doubts about the suitability of mannitol (which was previously feared to have deleterious effects on an already chemically compromised renal tubular epithelium) are no longer seriously considered. There is even some evidence that the use of mannitol may actually improve peritubular circulation. Many physicians favor the use of furosemide over mannitol as a drug that affords more concise control of the situation.

If renal failure results despite these measures, the patient may require maintenance by dialysis and the requisite support therapy provided by a specialized nephrology unit. Fortunately, the majority of these patients recover. A variable period of severe oliguria or anuria (several days to 3 weeks) may be followed in such cases by a brisk diuresis, and then by the gradual recovery of concentrating and diluting ability of the kidneys.

In certain selected cases of acute hemolytic transfusion reactions, transfusion with either therapeutic plasma exchange (TPE) or whole blood exchange has been considered. Typically, large amounts of incompatible blood have been administered or a large mass of circulating RBC stroma is present, especially where overt renal failure has not yet become established.[55] No statistics are currently available to support the ethicality of this procedure. It may nevertheless be considered in certain unique cases (eg, in a severe hemolytic crisis involving complications from acute autoimmune hemolytic anemia in which interruption of the hemolytic process, especially of continued complement activation, may be necessary to allow the transfusion of any cells to provide oxygen-carrying capacity sufficient for survival). In such cases, TPE using 5% human albumin or plasma protein fraction (which contains no complement components) may be an alternative consideration.

**Delayed Hemolytic Transfusion Reactions—Mechanism, Clinical, and Laboratory Recognition Management**

Delayed hemolytic reactions are generally caused by alloantibodies not detectable by antibody screening or crossmatch techniques performed at the time of transfusion. Most cases show a positive transfusion or obstetric history, in which 1 or both conditions have constituted a primary immunizing event to a blood group antigen not possessed by the patient and therefore absent from the RBCs. Such an event may lead to the priming of the immunologic memory of the recipient marked by a transient and clinically insignificant primary immune response in which small amounts of IgM antibody may have been formed that did not persist at a level detectable by ordinary blood bank techniques. A subsequent encounter with the same antigen (eg, by the transfusion of further RBCs bearing the antigen in question) will result in a secondary (anamnestic) response in which the immunologic memory of the patient may be triggered. The primed clone of B cells will then proliferate and begin to elaborate increasing amounts of IgG antibody specific to the antigen in question. As the antibody concentration increases, the transfused RBCs bearing the corresponding antigen (compatible with the patient's serum at the time of the initial crossmatch) will become increasingly incompatible as they are exposed to more and more IgG molecules. Over a period of several days, the RBCs will become increasingly labeled with antibody. If this is of subclass IgG3 or IgG1, varying degrees of complement activation may result. Most typically, however, partial activation of the complement pathway occurs, so that a significant residuum of cells labeled with C3d can thus be found in the circulation.[57,58]

Predominantly, the cells show an accelerated destruction rate, being sequestered by the macrophage system. On occasion, however, symptoms and signs similar to those of an acute immediate hemolytic reaction may occur. These reactions are symptomatically mild and may even be confined to the laboratory observation of a decrease in hematocrit corresponding to a transfused unit whose disappearance reactions—when they occur—usually do so within 2 weeks of the transfusion. Any reactions, however, may range from a few days to as long as 21 days posttransfusion.

Laboratory diagnosis of the delayed reaction depends on the demonstration of antibody on transfused RBCs, which generally will show a mixed-field reaction in the direct antiglobulin test. The patient's own native cells will not be antibody coated and therefore will not react with the Coombs' reagent. Conversely, the transfused cells that have acquired incompatibility anamnestically will react positively using this technique. The antibody can be identified by eluting it from these RBCs and testing it against appropriate panels of reagent RBCs of known antigenic composition.

Free antibody may now occur in the patient's plasma where none was detectable at the time of the original antibody screen or crossmatch. The specificity of this antibody, also determined by panel testing, should be identical to that of the antibody eluted from the donor cells. On occasion, routine testing fails to identify any specific alloantibody, although injection of small numbers of donor RBCs labeled with Cr51 may show accelerated removal of these cells. By the use of special techniques, including meticulous concentration methods, antibodies have been identified in a number of these cases.

Recognizable delayed transfusion reactions occur in about 1 in 5000 RBC (or whole blood) transfusions. These reactions are frequently asymptomatic or mild in nature, and seldom require any therapy other than careful monitoring of the patient in symptomatic cases. Sometimes it is necessary to retransfuse the patient if an administered unit is hemolyzed, and the anemia for which the unit was given requires correction. Generally, however, even in more severe delayed reactions, a life-threatening situation is seldom encountered. Irreversible renal damage is infrequent; in most cases, conservative therapy is all that is required. Should an exceptional case occur in which symptoms and signs become alarming, it may be necessary to follow the same principles of treatment used for an acute hemolytic transfusion reaction.

**Prevention of Hemolytic Transfusion Reactions**

Prevention of delayed hemolytic transfusion reactions is difficult. There is no way of predicting which patients have been sensitized to a given blood group antigen by previous transfusion or pregnancy. Where people have been multiply transfused, and especially those in whom 1 or more alloantibodies have been formed, it may be advisable to perform extended typing on the patient and to match phenotypically the patient's antigenic profile as closely as possible. This precaution is necessary to prevent further alloimmunization or anamnestic stimulation of a previous sensitization not yet manifested by the appearance of its corresponding antibody.

The overwhelming majority of acute hemolytic transfusion reactions result from human error. This usually involves the transfusion of the wrong unit to the wrong patient. Several measures are necessary to minimize this risk, although apparently nothing prevents it entirely. Some of these measures are as follows:

1) Meticulous labeling of the unit with positive patient identification data that should include the patient's first name, middle initial, last name, and hospital number, as well as all the requisite labeling required by the Food and Drug Administration (FDA) and by the American Association of Blood Banks (AABB). No unit should be issued for elective transfusion unless these data match exactly the data presented to the blood bank by the person collecting the unit. Two persons, the person collecting the unit and the blood bank technologist, should meticulously compare the identification data that each has, and only when these match in every respect should the unit be released. The release must be fully documented, and an appropriate person who is authorized by the hospital must sign for the unit.
2) Not more than 1 unit should be issued on a given patient at the same time unless special emergent clinical circumstances exist.
3) If units are to be issued at about the same time for more than 1 patient and in more than 1 location, they should not all be checked out to the same person. Otherwise, great opportunity exists for units to become mixed-up and inadvertently administered to the wrong person.
4) Before a transfusion is begun, 2 persons should be involved in the identification of a particular unit to the corresponding patient. Just as 2 persons were involved in checking out the unit from the blood bank, so 2 other persons (nurses, physicians, physicians' assistants) should be involved at the administrative end. Failure to follow this procedure meticulously also contributes measurably to the cause of serious transfusion reactions.
5) Meticulous records of the transfusion, together with appropriate and careful monitoring of the patient's vital signs, must be maintained on every transfusion.
6) Uncrossmatched units should only be released from the blood bank in major emergencies and only on receipt of a physician-signed release form. Such a precaution will protect the blood bank from legal liability for untoward effects of such uncrossmatched blood and justifies the use of such a product on the basis of serious and life-threatening clinical circumstances. Such blood should be group O, Rh-negative unless:
    a) The patient has been typed by the hospital blood bank during the current admission.
    b) Irrefutable identification data for the patient are present. Type-specific blood should never be issued uncrossmatched to a recipient, even in dire emergency, on the basis of blood type, blood type tattooed on the patient's body, etc. Such things have frequently been the cause of tragic error.

7) Wherever possible, an acceptable form of compatibility testing between the recipient's serum or plasma and the donor RBCs should be performed. This may be by 1 of the standard crossmatch procedures (as described in the *Technical Manual* of the AABB) or by an immediate-spin crossmatch between recipient serum and donor RBCs following careful screening of the recipient serum for irregular (allo-) antibodies. If the latter technique is used, the procedure should include at least 3 screening cells. This process will provide an adequate and fairly comprehensive range of blood group antigens and will minimize false negatives potentially resulting from dosage effects, sometimes seen where certain antigens are present only in the heterozygous state.

When carried out in this fashion, an in-depth antibody screen followed by a compatibility test for ABO seems to show no statistical difference in safety from the standard crossmatch procedure. Recently, a study exploring the possibility of replacing the immediate-spin crossmatch component of this procedure, which would bring about a "clerical match" between the 2 prior to releasing the units, indicated the small but significant frequency of clerical error. The study concluded that anything less than an antibody screen followed by an immediate-spin crossmatch may compromise safety.[59] The retention of at least this degree of compatibility testing would appear to correlate closely with maximum safety.

## Immunologic Reactions Involving Leukocytes

The frequency of nonhemolytic transfusion reactions, characterized by fever and shaking chills in patients with a history of previous transfusion or multiple pregnancy, has been recognized for many years. Similarly, the occurrence of agglutinating antibodies directed against leukocytes in multiply transfused patients is well known. The association between these findings (the dependency of febrile nonhemolytic transfusion reactions on the presence of leukoagglutinins) was described as early as 1957, and, since then, much has been learned regarding this etiologic relationship.[60-64] The association between noncardiogenic pulmonary edema and the presence of antileukocyte antibodies is also well established.[65-67]

### Pathogenesis of Leukocyte-Related Reactions

Antileukocyte antibodies, mostly IgG, are a frequent occurrence. These are the result of immunization, either by previous transfusion of leukocyte-containing blood products or of fetomaternal hemorrhages, with transfer of leukocyte antigen either during the third stage of labor or transplacentally during pregnancy, due to repeated minute placental separations occurring in the second and third trimesters. Immunizations to leukocyte antigens resulting from transfusion bear a direct relationship to transfusion frequency and exposure to leukocyte-containing products. Transfusion of 5 to 10 units of leukocyte-containing blood components frequently results in sensitization either to leukocyte-specific or HLA antigens, the appearance of leukoagglutinating or lymphocytotoxic antibodies, or both.[68-70] Patients who have had febrile transfusion reactions do not experience chills and fever when transfused with leukocyte-poor products (washed red blood, RBCs, or platelets), and even patients transfused with whole blood in which neutrophils but not lymphocytes were depleted have not experienced such reactions.[71] On the other hand, typical febrile reactions have been observed when granulocyte-depleted but lymphocyte-rich products have been transfused to a patient with antileukocyte antibodies.[72]

Fetomaternal hemorrhage occurring during the third stage of labor or transplacentally in the later stages of pregnancy is a common source of immunization to leukocyte antigens. Both leukoagglutinins and lymphocytotoxic anti-HLA antibodies are, therefore, common in multiparous women, and transfusion of leukocyte-containing blood products to such persons is likely to result in a febrile transfusion reaction. Conversely, the transfusion of blood products containing potent antileukocyte antibodies (especially leukoagglutinins) to other people may result in both a febrile response or in the development of significant pulmonary infiltrative reactions or noncardiogenic pulmonary edema.

Lymphocytotoxic antibodies (anti-HLA) resulting from immunization of women through fetomaternal hemorrhage also occur commonly after first pregnancies with incidences as high as 4% to 25% after first pregnancies and, in 55% or more cases, after the third pregnancy.[73-76] IgG leukoagglutinins directed against neutrophil-specific antigens may on occasion pass the placental barrier and produce immune neonatal neutropenia. Lymphocytotoxic antibodies directed against HLA antibodies, however, do not produce this effect since they appear to be absorbed out within the placenta.

The pathophysiology of leukocyte-related immune reactions is fairly simple. In the typical febrile reaction, transfusion of leukocyte-containing products into the recipient, whose plasma contains significant titers of leukoagglutinins, is followed by attachment of the antibody to corresponding receptors on leukocyte cell membranes. This action produces varying degrees of complement activation and complement-mediated leukoagglutination. Activation of the complement pathway will result in compromise of the cell membrane. This releases "androgenesis pyrogen" (including but not necessarily limited to interleukin I, IL-I), which stimulates the thermoregulatory center in the brain stem, producing a response similar to that that would be obtained by perfusing the center with blood at a lower-than-normal physiologic temperature. The result is an array of complex neuroendocrine, muscular, and cardiovascular response, the net effect of which is simultaneous heat conservation and increased heat production, with a sharp and abrupt rise in body temperature. Initially, peripheral vasoconstriction of cutaneous blood vessels induces pallor. Skin feels cold to the touch, but, because sweating is inhibited, it is also dry. At the same time, showers of uncoordinated motor impulses induce fibrillary contractions throughout the skeletal musculature, which creates the sensation of shivering, the phenomenon that is highly productive of heat. Thus, the combination of peripheral vasoconstriction, inhibition of sweating, and increased heat production through uncoordinated muscular activity results in a rapid rise of ambient body temperature. This characterizes the febrile response, which can be expected to continue as long as pyrogenic substances are being released from leukocytes (ie, as long as the thermal regulatory center continues to be stimulated by these substances). The reaction will subside when no further devitalization of leukocytes occurs, either because all transfused leukocytes have been compromised by circulating antibody within the recipient, or because passively transferred leukoagglutinin from a donor blood component has been completely consumed by interaction with the recipient's own leukocytes. At such a time, a defervescence occurs. The patient experiences a "flush," profuse sweating and subsidence of the fever. A typical attack begins some 30 minutes to 2 hours after beginning the transfusion and subsides variably over the next 2 to 24 hours.

Noncardiogenic pulmonary infiltrates or edema occasionally accompany severe leukocyte-associated reactions. This complication is most often seen with the transfusion of components containing high concentrations of leukoagglutinins in the donor plasma.[77] Although the reasons for these are somewhat obscure, one can speculate that these antibodies, delivered into a peripheral vein of plasma containing a high concentration of leukoagglutinin, might enter the pulmonary circulation relatively undiluted. Since pulmonary capillaries contain large numbers of marginated granulocytes, it follows that many of these cells will be promptly exposed to relatively high concentrations of antibody during the early stages of the transfusion. If the granulocytes happen to carry antigenic receptors corresponding to the antibodies transfused, then antibody binding and complement activation are likely to occur, with resulting cell membrane denaturation. Thus, a variety of intracellular products may be delivered rapidly into the pulmonary microcirculation. Some of these are likely to be vasoactive and result in pulmonary capillary vasodilatation with an increased capillary permeability. This will force seepage of plasma forced into the pulmonary interstitium and, ultimately, into alveolar spaces. The entire mechanism of such a sequence of events is not fully understood. It is known, however, that certain leukocyte-generated products (eg, leukotrienes) have a potent effect on the microcirculation of the lung and may be expected to generate an increase in capillary permeability.[1] Other vasoactive substances derived from aggregated and complement-devitalized leukocytes may include complement fragments (C3a, C5a, C5, 6, 7 complex), lysosomal enzymes, and superoxide anion. The combined effects of the release of such a complex of substances are capillary vasodilatation, endothelial cell injury, and significant increase in capillary permeability.

### Clinical Features

The typical febrile reaction usually begins relatively early in the transfusion process, frequently within the first half hour, but this may also be delayed for up to 2 hours. The patient complains of being cold or chilly, followed soon after by the onset of shaking chills that may be quite severe. These are soon followed by a rapid rise in temperature, generally of 2° to 3°C. The chills and fever are accompanied by varying degrees of tachycardia and, in more severe cases, dyspnea and cyanosis. Occasionally, some degree of hypotension may occur, but this is unusual. Most frequently, blood pressure shows no change. However, a transient rise, especially in systolic pressure, may be observed and probably correlates with catecholamine release from the adrenal medulla as a general stress-related phenomena.

In those cases complicated by noncardiogenic pulmonary edema, a picture of severe dyspnea with nonproductive cough, cyanosis, and pulmonary rales is superimposed on the features of a febrile reaction. Chest roentgenograms of such patients often show extensive lower-lobe infiltrates, often characterized by nodular perihilar shadows that tend to become confluent; these may extend more widely throughout the lung fields. In such cases, death from asphyxia is a real possibility. Although pulmonary infiltrates of minor degree are probably quite common in febrile reactions, life-threatening pulmonary edema is fortunately of rare occurrence. When it is observed, it constitutes a major medical emergency with the high potential for mortality.

### Laboratory Recognition

Febrile transfusion reactions are generally diagnosed clinically. In ordinary hospital circumstances, the laboratory contributes little information of diagnostic significance. However, shaking chills, fever, tachycardia, anxiety, and dyspnea are common symptoms and signs that can accompany a hemolytic transfusion reaction. Thus, simple laboratory tests should be routinely performed, including a direct antiglobulin test on the patient's RBCs and a screening of the patient's plasma for free hemoglobin. If the results of these 2 tests are negative, an acute hemolytic reaction can generally be excluded. The clinical features will then be ascribed to a leukocyte-related reaction.

Examination of the patient's plasma for leukoagglutinins and lymphocytotoxic antibodies may well be beyond the scope of an ordinary hospital laboratory, but may prove to be important for a patient who is likely to require repeated transfusion therapy in the future. However, with the advent of highly effective techniques for the preparation of leukocyte-poor components, including platelet concentrates, such testing procedures will be needed only infrequently.

### Management

The majority of febrile transfusion reactions, although often alarming, do not pose a significant threat to the patient. Symptomatic treatment with a suitable antipyretic agent and reassurance from the clinician are frequently all that is necessary. If the transfusion is still in progress when the reaction begins, it should be promptly discontinued, and, if further transfusion is necessary, a different unit should be given. The use of leukocyte-poor products for subsequent transfusions is recommended, since the majority of such reactions result from leukocyte-containing components. Aspirin, used as an antipyretic, is recommended for febrile transfusion reactions where no clinical contraindications exist. Since aspirin interferes with the creation of prostaglandin E1 synthesis in the cells of the thermoregulatory center, and the effective stimulation of these cells by pyrogens is in part mediated by prostaglandin, it is likely that the efficacy of aspirin as an antipyretic is related to this function.

Noncardiogenic pulmonary edema is a more difficult problem with which to deal. Where this condition generally constitutes a life-threatening emergency, the management of a fully developed attack is difficult. Steroids may produce a favorable response in treatment of this disorder, in that they may help to inhibit antigen-antibody interaction between leukoagglutinins and their corresponding antigenic receptors on granulocytes. However, they may also diminish superoxide anion synthesis.[78] Steroids should be given intravenously in large doses (eg, 30 mg/kg every 6 hours of dimethylprednisolone for up to 48 hours) to bring the condition under control.[79] In addition, the administration of oxygen, intravenous diuretics, and positive-pressure ventilation should be used according to the patient's clinical condition.

### Methods for Prevention

The use of leukocyte-poor blood or blood components constitutes a major advance in the prevention of febrile transfusion reactions, noncardiogenic pulmonary edema, and acquired refractoriness to transfused granulocytes and platelets.[80] The methods available for reducing the number of leukocytes in blood components include washing, glycerolizing, freezing, thawing, deglycerolizing (followed by washing), differential centrifugation, and filtration. The use of washed and frozen deglycerolized RBC concentrates has the advantage of removing not only leukocyte-related material and platelet-related material but also plasma, thereby eliminating substantial risk from both leukocyte-related and plasma-related transfusion reactions. Conversely, the cost of these procedures is significant and generally higher than that of filtration, while this process has the added disadvantage of sacrificing up to 20% of the RBCs that are lost in the washing process.

Currently, the most effective method for the removal of leukocytes is that of selective (leukocyte-specific) filtration.[81,82] Modern selective filters used for the trapping of leukocytes are distinct from microaggregate filters in this way: the removal of leukocytes is not dependent on pore size but, instead, relies on the use of a multilayered barrier-screen filter composed of a medium that selectively binds leukocytes while retaining only a minimum of other formed elements of blood. Such filters are currently available for whole blood, RBCs, and platelet concentrates. Their success, according to the manufacturer's reports, is indicated by an effectiveness rate exceeding 99%. This rate of success compares closely with frozen deglycerolized RBCs and is significantly superior to that of washed products. There is also a negligible loss of RBCs. Filters suitable for use with platelet concentrates are proving especially useful. It should be pointed out, however, that filters do not remove plasma, and therefore have no effect on the passive transfer of antileukocyte antibody that may be contained in some donor plasmas. Proper donor selectivity may therefore be a significant factor in eliminating this latter risk as far as possible.

## Immunologic Reactions Relating to Platelet Transfusion

### Alloimmunization and Refractoriness

The actual platelet count, which can be obtained by platelet transfusion, depends on a number of factors that must be taken into consideration before true refractoriness (ie, antibody-mediated removal of transfused platelets, which causes failure to increase platelet count after transfusion) is diagnosed. Factors to be considered are the following: 1) active bleeding with consumption of platelets; 2) the presence of splenomegaly, with nonimmunologic trapping of platelets in the enlarged spleen; 3) the presence of active infection or of inflammatory foci with augmented platelet consumption; and 4) the adequacy of dosage relative to the patient's blood volume.

In a nonbleeding patient, in whom the latter 3 of these factors can be reasonably excluded, the most likely explanation for failure to obtain a theoretic count increment after platelet transfusion is antibody-mediated refractoriness. This presupposes the presence of alloantibodies directed against platelets (ie, either against histocompatibility antigens or platelet-specific antigens) in the recipient's plasma. Of the 2, it is more likely that alloantibodies directed against histocompatibility antigens will be present to cause clinical refractoriness.[81]

Assume that the average platelet content of a unit-equivalent of platelet concentrate is $5 \times 10^{10}$, whether it is produced by centrifugal apheresis or by differential centrifugation of a single whole blood unit. If an 8-pack (8-unit equivalence) of apheresis-produced platelets were given, or 8 single-donor unit–derived platelet concentrates pooled into a single volume, platelet dosage should be nearly equivalent to a total dosage of $8 \times (5 \times 10^{10}) = 4 \times 10^{11}$ platelets.

If this total volume is delivered into a subject with a blood volume of about 5 L, then we might expect the theoretic count increment after transfusion to be:

$$CI = \frac{4 \times 10^{11}}{5 \times 10^{3} \times 10^{3}} \times 0.5 = 40{,}000/\mu L$$

The factor 0.5 in this equation is an empiric "fudge factor," based on the observation that counts of only 50% to 60% of the expected are generally observed. This difference most likely results from mechanical factors, such as physical damage or destruction of platelets at some point in the processing, loss by adhesion to the bag and tubing, adhesion to the filter, and mechanical removal, especially of damaged platelets, in vivo. Results a little higher or a little lower than this may be expected, but results conspicuously greater than this are unusual.

Posed differently, transfusion of a single platelet concentrate made from 1 unit of fresh whole blood may be expected to raise the platelet count of a nonbleeding person by about 8000/μL. Conspicuous failure to achieve such a result in the absence of the several nonimmune factors or in the absence of DIC is almost always an indication of antibody-mediated refractoriness. Under these circumstances, antiplatelet antibodies bring about a conspicuous shortening of the circulating life span of the platelets with rapid sequestration by the macrophage system. This common problem is most often observed in patients receiving multiple transfusions of platelet concentrates and is quite common. For example, a recipient receiving random pooled platelets derived from 10 to 20 different donors can be expected to show evidence of antibody-mediated refractoriness in about 2 weeks.[82] The antibodies formed in these circumstances are generally directed against HLA antigens not possessed by the recipient. This refractoriness may be temporarily short-lived. After an interval of a few weeks the patient may again show a moderate or "good" count increment after random platelet transfusion, since in the interim period antibody levels frequently decline to the point where platelets that would formerly have been vulnerable are now reasonably well tolerated. However, anamnestic stimulation of the immune system by such antigens will inevitably result in the return of refractoriness after further transfusion.[83]

It is well recognized that platelet refractoriness may also derive from alloimmunization of platelets by HLA antigen present on granulocytes and lymphocytes, in addition to platelets. Thus, it is highly desirable to use leukocyte-specific filtration of RBC or whole blood units for administration to people requiring repeated transfusion therapy. Alternately, saline-washed or frozen, deglycerolized, saline-suspended RBCs can also be used in these circumstances. Some evidence exists that the development of both leukoagglutinins and anti-HLA antibodies can be reduced even in repeated platelet therapy by the use of a selective leukocyte-specific filter designed for use with platelet concentrates, as distinct from RBCs.[84]

The problem of refractoriness can be addressed in 1 of 2 ways.

1) Platelets collected from donors whose lymphocytoxicity crossmatch is found to be compatible with the recipient's serum or plasma can be used. In this first instance, the anti-HLA antibodies in the recipient's serum are compatible with the lymphocytes of the prospective donor. Thus, by extrapolation, the same donor's platelets should also be compatible since the corresponding HLA antigens are clearly absent both from the donor's lymphocytes and platelets.[85]

2) Alternatively, platelet concentrates can be made from donors (usually siblings or first-order family members) whose HLA antigenic genotype is identical to or closely similar to that of the recipient.[86,87]

Again, patients showing sensitization to PLA1 may respond favorably to transfusion with platelets derived from donors shown to be negative for this antigen.[88] Regardless of the method used, however, locating a sufficient number of compatible platelet donors may require screening a significant number of persons. This may prove to be tedious and expensive. Where repeated platelet transfusions are a necessity, as for example in a patient at or approaching the nadir of leukemia chemotherapy, every effort should be made to find at least 2 or 3 donors so that a sufficient amount of platelets can be provided without subjecting any 1 donor to an unreasonable number of apheresis procedures.

Although platelets do carry ABH antigens, they do not display a high antigenic density for them. Transfusion of ABH-incompatible platelets will result in some diminished life span within the circulation, and count increments will be suboptimal in some cases. However, these effects are usually slight and many physicians believe them to be of no particular significance. It is generally recommended that platelets should be ABH-compatible with recipient plasma whenever possible. When only ABH-incompatible platelets are available and a genuine clinical need for transfusion of them exists, they should not be withheld.[89-91] By contrast, the Rh type of the platelet appears to have little significance for transfusion purposes, although platelet concentrates derived from Rh-positive donors should not be transfused to Rh-negative recipients, especially in female children or women of child-bearing age, since they may contain sufficient RBCs to bring about alloimmunization to Rho (D).

### Febrile Transfusion Reactions

The relatively common occurrence of febrile transfusion reactions, as described in relation to leukocytes, with the use of platelet concentrates is most easily explained by the fact that platelet concentrates are heavily contaminated with leukocytes. Moreover, the occurrence of leukocyte-mediated febrile transfusion reactions in association with platelet concentrates appears to limit the effectiveness and adequacy of the count increment in such circumstances.[92] The recent introduction of leukocyte-specific filters usable with platelet concentrates is likely to eliminate much of this problem.[84,93]

### Immune Neonatal Thrombocytopenia

Passive transfer of antiplatelet antibodies across the placental barrier from maternal plasma to the fetal circulation may sometimes result in immune-mediated thrombocytopenia developing in the infant. This may be due to transfer of IgG autoantibody with antiplatelet specificity in pregnant women who have autoimmune thrombocytopenia (ATP, ITP). A few cases are due to the immunization of the mother to a platelet-specific antigen that she does not herself possess but that is present on her infant's platelets. Exposure to such antigens may lead to her alloimmunization in a manner directly analogous to the mechanism by which hemolytic disease of the newborn is obtained (ie, with RBC antigens). In an overwhelming majority of cases, the antibody involved is anti-$Pl^{A1}$. This is in spite of the fact that, even though the corresponding antigen is of high incidence, the antibody is present in about 98% of the random population.[94,95]

A brief summary of our current understanding of platelet-specific antigens is given in Table 4-4. Several "platelet group" systems are recognized. In most of these, at least 2 alleles are identified, usually 1 of much higher incidence than the other; in 2 of the systems, only 1 has been identified in each case. Although of high incidence, $Pl^{A1}$ is by far the most potent of the identified platelet-specific antigens. Frequently, the small proportion of people who are negative for this antigen exhibit the corresponding antibody in their plasma, even with a noncontributory transfusion or obstetric history. Therefore, it is usual for children (fetuses, prenates, or neonates) in the course of a first pregnancy to be affected. Also, some of these cases may represent genuine alloimmunization by minor degrees of fetomaternal hemorrhage occurring in the later stages of pregnancy. In any case, when the fetus possesses the corresponding antigen, anamnestic increases in maternal antibody titer are the rule in late pregnancy, and the infant can be expected to show parallel increases in antigen level. Although the condition is often mild and self-limiting, some severe examples of thrombocytopenia may occur, characterized by extensive bruising. A significant risk of intracranial hemorrhage is occasionally encountered, especially when multiply successive pregnancies have resulted in higher antibody titers. If such a situation is encountered, the infant should be transfused with maternal platelets that are cautiously washed or packed. The maternal plasma should be expressed and replaced with an equal volume of homologous plasma (group AB) to eliminate maternal antibody. Where a severe problem has occurred once, it may be advisable to consider delivery by cesarean section in later pregnancies. This process should be initiated at about 36 weeks' gestation to avoid the period of greatest antibody transfer, which is the latter part of the third trimester of pregnancy. The mother, in this instance, may electively donate platelets on the day preceding the operation to be used as described should the infant require them.

### Posttransfusion Purpura

Posttransfusion purpura (PTP) is a rare complication found overwhelmingly among recipients of blood transfusions whose platelets lack the $Pl^{A1}$

**TABLE 4-4 | PRINCIPAL PLATELET-SPECIFIC ANTIGENIC SYSTEMS**

| System | Antigens | New Designation | Phenotype Frequency (%) | Glycoprotein Fraction |
|---|---|---|---|---|
| Plp | $Pl^{A1}(Zw^{a})$ | HPA-1a | 97.6 | IIIa |
| | $Pl^{A2}(Zw^{b})$ | HPA-1b | 26.2 | IIIa |
| Ko | $(S1b^{a})$ | HPA-2b | 14.3 | Ib |
| | $Ko^{b}$ | HPA-2b | 99.4 | Ib |
| $Ba^{k}$ | $Ba^{ka}$ | HPA-3a | 86.7 | IIb |
| | $Ba^{kb}$ | HPA-3b | 63.8 | IIb |
| $Yu^{k}$ | $Yu^{ka}$ | HPA-4b | <0.1 | IIIa |
| | $Yu^{kb}$ | HPA-4a | 99.9 | IIIa |
| Br | $Br^{a}$ | HPA-5b | 20.0 | Ia |
| | $Br^{b}$ | HPA-5a | 99.1 | Ia |
| $Na^{k}$ | $Na^{ka}$ | — | ? | IV |

antigen. On the uncommon occasions when it is observed, it seems to appear within a week or so of the receipt of blood transfusions and may persist anywhere from a few days to as long as 2 months.[96-103] In most documented cases, anti-$Pl^{A1}$ alloantibody is present in the patient's plasma. The majority of cases have occurred in middle-aged to elderly women with a history of multiparity, with or without a positive transfusion history. Less commonly, the condition has been observed without a positive obstetric history but with a history of previous blood transfusions. Isoimmunization (the occurrence of apparently "naturally occurring" antibodies) may be noted without either a positive transfusion or obstetric history. On occasion the condition has developed following a first experience with transfusion of blood products,[104,105] and is characterized by the onset of severe, even catastrophic, thrombocytopenia beginning several days after the transfusion with blood products, frequently complicated by cutaneous and mucosal hemorrhage, which may be severe and sometimes even life threatening. Marked degrees of thrombocytopenia may occur with platelet counts of less than 5000/µL and with all the attendant risks of severe mucosal or central nervous system hemorrhage that this entails.

The mechanism by which an alloantibody ostensibly compatible with the patient's autologous platelets is able to bring about an apparently paradoxic decrease in the circulating number of these platelets, after transfusion with other blood products, is not fully understood. The patient's own platelets are diminished, rather than those of a transfused product. Transfusion of blood products containing $Pl^{A1}$ antigen, either on the surface of platelet fragments in stored products or solubilized in the plasma, generates immune complexes in large quantities within the recipient's plasma. These are capable of binding nonspecifically to the recipient's platelets to bring about their sequestration by the macrophage system.[101,102] In these circumstances, the patient's own platelets are trapped fortuitously by the familiar "innocent bystander" mechanism, frequently seen as a complication of disorders involving immune complex formation.

Treatment of these patients can be difficult. Steroid therapy, while advocated by some physicians, appears to be only marginally effective in most cases. Likewise, platelet transfusions with random-donor platelets are strongly contraindicated, because the transfused platelets will be rapidly destroyed, thereby further exacerbating the situation.[106] It is not likely that transfusion with $Pl^{A1}$-negative platelets will offer any particular advantage at this stage.[107] Better results are obtained with therapeutic plasma exchange or exchange transfusion where feasible.[97,99,100] The use of high-dose preparations of human immunoglobulin (eg, sandoglobulin) may also be useful in some cases.[108]

The frequency of $Pl^{A1}$-negative persons in our "lay population" and the observed infrequency of PTP are somewhat difficult to reconcile. It could well be that a significant number of unrecognized cases occur, whether uncomplicated by detectable clinical manifestations or with mild ones that are relatively easy to overlook. The literature, however, shows a surprisingly small number of cases.

### Passive Transfer of Antiplatelet Antibodies

Thrombocytopenia that results from the transfusion of recipients with blood products derived from persons who have circulating antiplatelet antibodies appears to be a rare occurrence. However, it has been demonstrated experimentally with anti-$Pl^{A1}$, anti-$PL^{A2}$, and autoantibodies occurring in idiopathic thrombocytopenia.[109,110] Ordinarily, persons likely to have such antibodies in their plasma would seldom be accepted as donors under modern screening criteria.

## Immunologic Reactions Associated With Immunoglobulins and Other Plasma-borne Antigens

### Immunoglobulin-Related Reactions and Side Effects of Intravenous Immunoglobulin Therapy

Some adverse reactions, variable in nature and severity, have been associated with sensitization of a person whose heavy chain–specific antigenic determinants of IgG (Gm) will generate consequent antibody formation. The initial immunizing event may be either exposure to blood products through transfusion, passive immunization, or pregnancy (fetomaternal hemorrhage). Such immunization frequently has been described following multiple transfusions for chronic anemia, hemoglobinopathies, multiple pregnancies following exchange transfusion for hemolytic disease of the newborn, or neonatal respiratory distress syndrome.[111-113] Large or multiple exposures to plasma protein–containing material seem to be required for immunization. Generally, single or infrequent administration of plasma protein products is not generally followed by sensitization.[114] Again, a small percentage of the population has hereditary deficiencies of some immunoglobulin subclasses, most often IgG2 or IgG4. Exposure to protein-containing blood products, especially when frequently repeated or after multiple pregnancies, may result in the formation of antibodies directed against these deficiencies.

Despite the relative frequency of anti-Gm antibodies, the administration of plasma protein–containing blood products infrequently leads to obvious adverse reactions in the recipient. Where these have occurred, the degree of severity has been highly variable, ranging from mild febrile-type responses, somewhat similar to those seen in leukocyte-associated reactions, to more significant allergic or anaphylactoid reactions including urticaria, giant urticaria, glottideal edema, hypotension, and shock.

The advent of intravenous therapy with high-dose administration of immunoglobulin has led to fairly common adverse reactions of varying severity. Most of these appear to result from the generation or release of vasoactive mediators, which in turn result from the formation of IgG aggregates in vivo or even from immune complexes generated by interaction of injected IgG with other immunoglobulin molecules, which have an antigenic specificity complementary to certain of the IgG molecules administered. Reactions of this type may be quite dramatic and include flushing, substernal oppression, feelings of acute anxiety or impending doom, tachycardia, and hypotension that might be severe and lead to actual shock.[115,116] In modern intravenous immunoglobulin preparations, aggregated IgG is present in only very low concentration. Thus, reactions of this type, which were observed with earlier preparations, are now uncommon. They are seldom seen with other immunoglobulin-containing preparations, such as anti-Rho (D) immune globulin or various commercial gamma globulin preparations for intramuscular or intravenous use.

Fortunately, genuine anaphylactic reactions are of uncommon occurrence. These are frequently associated with hereditary IgA deficiency, which may present major medical emergencies with potential for fatal results unless treated with great promptness. However, hereditary IgA deficiency is more common than was formerly believed. This condition probably occurs in about 1 out of 850 subjects in the random population.[117-119] About 1 in 4 of these persons may possess antibodies directed against IgA that appear to be "naturally occurring," since the persons concerned may not admit to any positive transfusion or obstetric history. In some cases, although not often, 1 or more exposures to blood products (including immunoglobulin administration) or 1 or more pregnancies may have occurred. Most IgA antibodies found in these cases are IgG in character.[120,121] Anti-IgA antibodies found in such subjects are generally class-specific, and they react with all varieties of IgA, including IgA myeloma paraprotein.[122]

The administration of even very small amounts of IgA-containing material either intravenously or intramuscularly to patients with IgA deficiency, who also have anti-IgA antibodies, almost invariably results in a severe and life-threatening anaphylactic reaction. The patient becomes flushed and manifests acute restlessness, anxiety, dizziness, disorientation, severe substernal discomfort, freezing, and severe dyspnea, followed quickly by laryngeal edema and circulatory collapse with profound hypotension. Confluent urticaria and giant urticaria are frequent concomitants.[123-127] There appears to be a direct relationship between antibody titer and severity of response: when the anti-IgA titer does not exceed 1:256, severe reactions appear to be infrequent.[128]

Promptness of treatment generally determines the patient's likelihood of survival. Administration of all blood product–containing material should cease immediately, and the condition should be treated with intravenous epinephrine, bronchodilators, oxygen, and intravenous fluids. Subsequently, after recovery and after a suitable time interval to allow for dissipation of administered plasma protein, the patient should be thoroughly examined for immunoglobulin status, including immunoelectrophoresis for the plasma to determine the presence or absence of IgA. The plasma should also be screened for IgA antibodies. If found, these should be quantitated. It may be useful to examine other members of the patient's family to demonstrate the genetic trait more accurately. The patient should be informed of the options available to correct this condition and of the extreme risk that he or she would undergo if exposed to the indiscriminate use of any further blood-derived product.

Clearly, a patient who is IgA deficient and possesses anti-IgA antibodies is in a singularly difficult dilemma if transfusion therapy is required. As a general rule, such patients may not be given any product containing plasma protein, unless it can be guaranteed that the product contains no IgA. If a patient requires RBC transfusions, frozen, deglycerolized, saline-suspended RBCs can generally be given safely, with little or no risk of reaction.[129] The use of simple washed RBC concentrates is not advised: a single-volume wash will not guarantee the complete absence of IgA, and a 2-volume wash is extremely wasteful of RBCs.

Antibodies directed against specific subclasses of IgA are occasionally encountered in patients whose total IgA as determined by quantitative measurement is not diminished.[130] Immunization to the missing subclasses is most often caused by previous transfusion and possibly by pregnancy. Rarely does antibody formation against the missing subclasses appear to be spontaneous. Such IgA antibodies of limited (subclass) specificity are likely to be encountered in multiply transfused individuals. For example, such antibodies have been encountered in as many as 4% of hemophiliacs. Often and most interestingly, they have appeared in the great majority of patients who have exhibited urticarial or other anaphylactoid transfusion reactions.[131] Reactions in these cases are of variable severity and anaphylactoid in nature, varying from simple urticaria to confluent urticaria with asthma, giant urticaria, laryngeal edema, and finally full-blown anaphylaxis. The latter, however, is much less frequent than in hereditary agammaglobulinemia-a. These reactions generally respond satisfactorily to administration of simple antihistamines, usually given by intramuscular injection. Occasionally, more severe reactions will require the use of epinephrine.

Whenever such an "allergic" reaction is observed, transfusion of the product concerned should be stopped, the patient's physician immediately notified, and an antihistamine administered intramuscularly. Rapid subsidence of the reaction within 20 minutes of the antihistamine injection may permit cautious restarting of the infusion. If any signs or symptoms recur, the product should be discontinued immediately. In subsequent transfusions, it may be prudent to consider administering an antihistamine prophylactically at the beginning of the procedure. Where possible (eg, in the case of RBC transfusions) washed or frozen, deglycerolized, saline-suspended RBCs should be used.

No patient can be specifically identified as having hereditary agammaglobulinemia-a. Transfusion with any product containing plasma protein, however small in amount, poses a serious problem with a high potential risk of anaphylactic reaction. National rare donor files contain lists of donors who are also deficient in IgA, and when possible and when time permits it may be necessary use blood derived from such donors for the specific transfusion of patients of this type. In emergencies, when such blood cannot be readily obtained and when transfusion of both RBCs and adequate volume is clinically necessary, frozen, deglycerolized saline-suspended RBCs or thoroughly washed RBC suspensions may be used in conjunction with non–plasma protein–containing colloidal solutions such as hydroxyethyl starch (Volex) as a plasma substitute.

Small concentrations of anti-IgM antibodies of limited specificity and frequently of low temperature optimum or thermal range occur in some 2% to 3% of donor blood.[132] Their occurrence in multiply transfused persons and in multiparous women is significantly higher, 7% to 21% and 4% to 8%, respectively.[133,134] Under normal clinical conditions, these antibodies do not seem to produce adverse transfusion reactions. However, patients with IgM paraprotein with rheumatoid factor activity sometimes react adversely to immunoglobulin infusion, which may result in acute cryoglobulinemia.[135]

IgE-mediated "allergic" reactions are among the most commonly observed adverse manifestations of transfusion of blood products. Most frequently, they show up as urticarial reactions of varying severity (eg, crops of "hives" breaking out on the skin and apparently migrating from 1 body part to the next) or in more severe examples that develop in multiple sites over a short period of time. Sometimes the lesions become confluent, and at other times giant urticaria combines with edema involving subcutaneous as well as superficial cutaneous structures. In the most severe cases, bronchospasm, laryngeal edema, airway obstruction, and all the manifestations of actual anaphylaxis may occur. In general, however, the overwhelming number of these reactions are mild, self-limited, and easily controllable by discontinuation of the transfusion together with administration of an antihistamine. Similar reactions may be observed in patients with antibodies directed against specific IgA subclasses. Laboratory investigation of these cases frequently presents no useful result. Occasionally, elevated plasma IgE titers are observed, but most often they are not. Moreover, the offending antigen is generally impossible to define. For example, few cases may be traced to food allergies. A patient having been sensitized to shrimp protein who receives a plasma-containing product from a donor who had recently ingested shrimp may experience a reaction of varying severity due to the interaction of passively transferred shrimp antigen, complexing with IgE anti-shrimp protein antibody. Localization of such immune complexes on mast cells will result in the liberation of histamine and other vasoactive mediators whose combined effects manifest the reaction.

Generally, the administration of an antihistamine (eg, 50 mg of diphenhydramine hydrochloride, Benadryl) intramuscularly promptly controls any symptoms and signs of an allergic reaction. As soon as the adverse effect is observed, the infusion of the blood product should be terminated. In these circumstances, and uniquely to this type of reaction, the component may be left hanging and reinfusion may be cautiously restarted if symptoms and signs rapidly subside after the administration of antihistamine. The subsequent reinfusion should be given slowly, and the patient should be carefully and constantly monitored. Any recurrence of adverse symptoms or signs (urticaria, itching or burning sensations, wheezing, etc) should cause the infusion to be instantly and permanently terminated. In such cases, it is advisable to use washed or frozen, deglycerolized products for future transfusions whenever possible.

### The Role of Lipoprotein Antigens

About 10 antigenic determinants (Ag) through low-density lipoproteins have been described and defined by antibodies specific to them.[136-139] Precipitating antibodies with various Ag specificities have been identified in the plasma of multiparous women and multiply transfused persons. Although febrile-type reactions have been observed with the transfusion of plasma-containing products to patients shown to have anti-Ag antibodies, a causal relationship between these antibodies and the transfused products has not been clearly demonstrated. It is perhaps more likely that the febrile responses observed were due to leukocyte antibodies rather than to lipoprotein antibodies.

## References

1. Anstall HB. Adverse reactions to transfusion. In: A Manual of Hemotherapy. New York, NY: John Wiley and Sons, Inc; 1984:362-365.
2. Anstall HB. Adverse reactions to transfusion. In: A Manual of Hemotherapy. New York, NY: John Wiley and Sons, Inc; 1984:327-328.
3. Engelfriet EP, van den Borne AECK, Beckers D, et al. Immune destruction of red cells. In: Immune-Mediated Cell Destruction. Arlington, Va: American Association of Blood Banks; 1981:93.
4. Issitt PD. Antibodies active at 30°C, room temperature, and below. In: Bulik S, ed. Clinically Significant and Insignificant Antibodies. Arlington, Va: American Association of Blood Banks; 1979:26.

5. Mollison PL, Cutbush M. The use of isotope-labeled red cells to determine incompatibility in vivo. Lancet. 1955;1:115.
6. Barton JC. Noninfectious transfusion reactions. In: Dutcher JP, ed. Modern Transfusion Therapy. Boca Raton, Fla: CRC Press, Inc; 1990:57-92.
7. Cutbush M, Mollison PL. Relation between characteristics of blood group antibodies in vitro and associated patterns of red cell destruction in vivo. Br J Haematol. 1958;4:115.
8. Davey RJ. Mechanisms of premature red cell destruction. In: Judd JW, Barnes A, eds. Clinical and Serological Aspects of Transfusion Reactions: A Technical Workshop. Arlington, Va: American Association of Blood Banks; 1982:3.
9. Mollison PL. Factors determining the selective clinical importance of different blood-group antibodies. Br Mem Ed Bull. 1959;15:92.
10. Mollison PL, Johnson CA, Prior DM. Dose-related destruction of A1-cells by anti-A1. Vox Sang. 1978;35:149.
11. Mascouredis SD, Sudora EJ, Mahan L, et al. Antigen site-densities and ultrastructural distribution pattern of IH red cell antigens. Transfusion. 1976;16:94.
12. Petz LD, Garritty G. Acquired Immune Hemolytic Anemia. New York, NY: Churchill-Livingstone; 1980:64.
13. Sherman SP, Taswell HS. The need for saline-washed red blood cells in paroxysmal nocturnal hemoglobinuria. Transfusion. 1977;17:68.
14. Jankins DE. Paroxysmal nocturnal hemoglobinuria hemolytic systems. In: CA Bell, ed. Seminar on the Laboratory Management of Hemolysis. Arlington, Va: American Association of Blood Banks; 1979:45.
15. Nunn LD, Chaplin H. Rosette formation by sensitized human red cells: effects of source of peripheral leukocyte macrophages. Vox Sang. 1977;33:129.
16. Packer JJ, Greendyke RN, Swisher SN. The inhibition of erythrophagocytosis in vitro by corticosteroids. Trans Assoc Am Physicians. 1960;73:93.
17. Lawley TJ, Hill RP, Gaoli AS, et al. Defective Fc receptor functions associated with HLA-D8/DRw haplotype. N Engl J Med. 1981;304:185.
18. Williams BD, Lockwood CN, Russell BA, et al. Deficient reticuloendothelial system function in rheumatoid arthritis. Lancet. 1979;1:1311.
19. Frank MM, Hamburger NJ, Lawley TJ, et al. Defective reticuloendothelial system Fc receptor response in disseminated lupus erythematosus. N Engl J Med. 1979;300:518.
20. Greenwalt TJ. Pathogenesis and management of hemolytic transfusion reactions. Semin Hematol. 1981;18:84.
21. Mollison PL. Red cell incompatibility in vivo. In: Blood Transfusion in Clinical Medicine. 7th ed. Oxford: Blackwell Scientific; 1983:chap 1-2.
22. Ebert RE, Emerson CT. A clinical study of transfusion reactions. The hemolytic effect of group O blood and blood plasma containing incompatible isoagglutinins. J Clin Invest. 1946;25:627.
23. Anstall HB. Adverse reactions to transfusion. A Manual of Hemotherapy. New York, NY: John Wiley & Sons, Inc; 1984:364.
24. Wiener AS, Maloney WC. Hemolytic transfusion reactions, IV: differential diagnosis, "dangerous universal donor," or intragroup incompatibility. Am J Clin Pathol. 1943;18:74.
25. Delmas-Marsalet Y, Parquet-Gernec A, Bauters S, et al. Anénies Hémolytiques dues à la plasma therapie shez les hemopiles. Rev Fr Transfusion. 1969;12:351.
26. Imwood MJ, Zuliani B. Anti-A hemolytic transfusion with packed O cells. Ann Intern Med. 1978;89:51.
27. Zoes C, Dube EV, Miller HJ, et al. Anti-A in the plasma of platelet concentrates causing a hemolytic reaction. Transfusion. 1977;17:29.
28. Siber GR, Ambrosino DM, Gorgone BC. Blood group A-like substance in a preparation of pneumococcal vaccine. Ann Intern Med. 1982;96:580.

29. Pierce RN, Reich LOM, Meyer K. Hemolysis following platelet transfusions from ABO-incompatible donors. Transfusion. 1985;25:60.
30. Gasser C. Akute hämolytische Krisen nach Plasma-transfusionen. Helv Paediatr Acta. 1935;1:38.
31. Stevens AR, Finch CA. A dangerous universal transfusion of group O blood. Am J Clin Pathol. 1954;24:612.
32. Topley E, Bull JP, Maycock WD, et al. The relation of the isoagglutinins in pooled plasma to the hemolytic anemia of burns. J Clin Pathol. 1963;16:79.
33. Keidan SE, Loboar E, Mainwaring D. Acute anemia in a hemophiliac due to transfusion of incompatible plasma. Lancet. 1966;1:179.
34. Rossati LA, Barnes B, Oberman H, et al. Hemolytic anemia due to anti-A in concentrated anti-hemophilic factor preparations. Transfusion. 1979;10:139.
35. Tamagani GP, Dormandy KKM, Ellis D, et al. Factor VIII concentrate in hemophilia (letter). Lancet. 1975;2:188.
36. Brox AG, Cournoyer D, Sternback M, et al. Hemolytic anemia following intravenous gammaglobulin administration. Am J Med. 1987;82:633.
37. Schmuck K. Cited in Mollison PL: Hemolytic transfusion reactions. In: Blood Transfusion in Clinical Medicine. 75th ed. Oxford: Blackwell Scientific; 1983:636.
38. Hows J, Beddow K, Gordon-Smith E, et al. Donor-derived red cell antibodies and hemolysis after allogenic bone marrow transplantation. Blood. 1986;67:177.
39. Haas RJ, Rieber P, Helmig M, et al. Acquired immune hemylosis by anti-A1 antibody following bone marrow transplantation. Blut. 1986;53:401.
40. Evans RE, Turner E, Bingham M. Tv resistance of C prime 142-coated cells to complement hemolysis by cold agglutinin. Stockholm: Proceedings of the Tenth Congress of the International Society of Blood Transfusion; 1964-5:834.
41. Crosby WH, Steffanini M. Pathogenesis of the plasma transfusion reaction with special reference to the blood coagulation system. J Lab Clin Med. 1952;40:374.
42. Burn FH, Esham WT, Bull RW. The significance of hemoglobulinuria and associated hemosiderinuria. J Exp Med. 1969;129:909.
43. Crosby WH, Dameshek W. The significance of hemoglobinuria and hemosiderinuria with particular reference to different types of hemolytic anemia. J Lab Clin Med. 1951;38:3.
44. Barton JC. Noninfectious transfusion reactions. In: Dutcher JP, ed. Modern Transfusion Therapy. Boca Raton, Fla: CRC Press; 1990:60.
45. Luke RG, Linton AL, Briggs JD, et al. Mannitol therapy in acute renal failure. Lancet. 1985;1:980.
46. Goldfinger D. Acute hemolytic transfusion reactions: a fresh look at pathogenesis and considerations regarding therapy. Transfusion. 1977;17:85.
47. Pineda AA, Brzica SN, Taswell HF. Hemolytic transfusion reaction: recent experience in a large blood bank. Mayo Clin Proc. 1978;53:378.
48. Mollison PL. Blood Transfusion in Clinical Medicine. 7th ed. Oxford: Blackwell Scientific; 1983:51.
49. Goldfinger D. Complications of hemolytic transfusion reactions: pathogenesis and therapy. In: New Approaches to Transfusion Reactions: A Technical Workshop. Arlington, Va: American Association of Blood Banks; 1974:15-38.
50. Henderson RS, Beattie TI, Kennedy AC. Dopamine-hydrochloride in oliguric states. Lancet. 1980;2:827.
51. Goldfinger D. Adverse reactions to blood transfusions. In: Mayer K, ed. Guidelines to Transfusion Practice. Arlington, Va: American Association of Blood Banks; 1980:137-154.
52. Barnes A. Complications of transfusions. In: Barnes A, Nelson IS, eds. Safe Transfusions: A Technical Workshop. Arlington, Va: American Association of Blood Banks; 1981:63-76.

53. Huestis DW, Bowe JR, Busch S. Practical Blood Transfusion. 3rd ed. Boston: Little, Brown and Co; 1981.
54. Greenwalt TJ. Pathogenesis as a management of hemolytic transfusion reactions. Semin Hematol. 1981;19:84.
55. Barry KG, Crosby WH. The prevention and treatment of renal failure following hemolytic transfusion reactions. Transfusion. 1963;3:34.
56. Holland PH. Other adverse effects of transfusion. In: Petz LD, Swisher SN, eds. Clinical Practice of Blood Transfusion. New York, NY: Churchill-Livingstone; 1981:288.
57. Salaman A, Mueller-Eckhardt C. Delayed hemolytic transfusion reactions: evidence for complement activation involving allogenic and autologous red cells. Transfusion. 1984;24:188.
58. Chaplain H. The implication of re-cell bound complement in delayed hemolytic transfusion reactions (editorial). Transfusion. 1984;24:185.
59. Shulman IA, Kent D. Safety in transfusion practice: is it safe to eliminate the major crossmatch for selected patients? Pathol Lab Med. 1989;113:270.
60. Dausset J, Neena A. Presence d'une leuco-agglutinine dans le serum d'un cas d'agrnulocytose chronique. C R Soc Biol (Paris). 1952;146:1532.
61. Goudsmit R, van Loughem JJ. Studies on the occurrence of leukocyte-antibodies. Vox Sang. 1953;3:58.
62. Miescher P, Fauconnet M. Mic en évidence de differents groupes leucocytaires shez l'homme. Schweiz Med Wochenschr. 1954;84:597.
63. van Loghem JJ, Sauer AJ, van der Hart M, et al. Zeldzane immunologische afwigkingen orozak van blood-transfusien reacties bij een lijder aan verwzoren hämolytische anemie. Med Tidschrf Geneesk. 1956;100:314.
64. Brittingham E, Chaplain H. Febrile transfusion reactions caused by sensitivity to donor leukocytes and platelets. JAMA. 1957;165:819.
65. Wolf CSW, Canale VC. Fatal pulmonary hypersensitivity reaction to HLA-incompatible blood transfusion: report of the case and review of the literature. Transfusion. 1976;16:135.
66. Kernoff PB, Durrant IJ, Rizza GR, et al. Severe allergic pulmonary edema after plasma transfusion. Br J Haematol. 1972;23:722.
67. Lalezari P, Radel E. Neutrophil-specific antigens: immunology and significance. Semin Hematol. 1974;11:281.
68. Levernz S, Ihle R, Frick G. HLA-system und Transfusion-reaktionen, I: Mitteilung. Dtsch Ges-Wesen. 1974;29:1546.
69. Levernz S, Ihle R, Frick G. HLA-system und Transfusion-reaktionen, II: Mitteilung. Dtsch Ges-Wesen. 1975;30:1688.
70. Pretty HM, Fudenberg HH, Perkins HA, et al. Anti-gammaglobulin antibodies after open heart surgery. Blood. 1968;32:205.
71. Greenwalt TJ, Gajewski M, McKenna JL. A new method for preparing buffy-coat poor blood. Transfusion. 1962;2:221.
72. Perkins HA, Payne R, Ferguson J, et al. Nonhemolytic febrile transfusion reactions: quantitative effect of blood components with emphasis on isoantigenic incompatibility of leukocytes. Vox Sang. 1966;11:578.
73. Goodman HS, Masaitis L. Analysis of isoimmune response to leucocytes, I: maternal cytotoxic leukocyte isoantibodies formed during the first pregnancy. Vox Sang. 1967;16:97.
74. Overwegg J, Engelfriet C. Cytotoxic leukocyte isoantibodies formed during the first pregnancy. Vox Sang. 1974;27:322.
75. Ahrons S. HLA antibodies: influence on the human fetus. Tissue Antigens. 1971;1:121.

76. Nymand G. Complement-fixing and lymphotoxic antibodies in serum of pregnant women at delivery. Vox Sang. 1974;27:322.

77. Grant RT, Perry S. The use of 51-chromium in the study of leukocyte kinetics in chronic myelocytic leukemia. J Lab Clin Med. 1968;71:614.

78. Shaden A. Methylprednisolone: traumacologic doses in shock lung syndrome. J Thorac Cardiovasc Surg. 1976;71:800.

79. Jacob HS, Craddock PR, Hammerschmidt DE, et al. Complement-induced granulocyte agglutination. N Engl J Med. 1980;302:789.

80. Polesky HF. The Emily Cooley Lecture. Leukocyte-poor blood: a study in the evolution of component therapy. In: Seminar and Blood Components. Arlington, Va: American Association of Blood Banks; 1977.

81. Hirsch FO, Gardner FH. The transfusion of human blood platelets. J Lab Clin Med. 1952;39:56.

82. van Rood JJ. Leukocyte grouping and organ transplantation. Br J Haematol. 1969;16:211.

83. Gockeman JP, Bowman RP, Conrad ME. Detection of platelet isoantibodies by 3H serotonin platelet release and its clinical application to the problem of platelet matching. J Clin Invest. 1975;55:75.

84. Treadwell F. Personal communication, 1991.

85. Vanke RA, Grunnet FC, Rogentine GN. Platelet transfusion therapy: the selection of compatible platelet donors for refractory patients by lymphocyte HLA typing. N Engl J Med. 1969;281:208.

86. Schiffer CA, Keller C, Dutcher JP, et al. Potential HLA-matched platelet donor availability for alloimmunized patients. Transfusion. 1983;23:286.

87. Lohrman HP, Bull MI, Decter JA, et al. Platelet transfusions from HLA-compatible donors to alloimmunized patients. Am Med. 1974;80:9.

88. Duquesnoy RJ, Fillip DJ, Aster RH. Influence of HLA-A2 on the effectiveness of platelet transfusions in alloimmunized thrombocytopenic patients. Blood. 1977;50:407.

89. Gurevitch J, Nelken D. ABO groups in blood platelets. J Lab Clin Med. 1954;44:562.

90. Slichter SJ. Mechanisms and management of platelet refractoriness. In: Nance ST, ed. Transfusion Medicine in the 1990s. Arlington, Va: American Association of Blood Banks; 1990.

91. Aster RH. Effect of anticoagulant and ABO incompatibility on recovery of transfused human platelets. Blood. 1965;26:732.

92. Herzog RH, Herzog GP, Bull MI, et al. Correction of poor platelet transfusion responses with leukocyte-poor HLA-matched platelet concentrates. Blood. 1975;46:743.

93. Schiffer CA, Hogge DF, Aisner J, et al. High-dose intravenous gammaglobulin in alloimmunized platelet transfusion recipients. Blood. 1984;64:937.

94. Shulman NR, Marder VJ, Hiller MC, et al. Platelet and leukocyte isoantigens and antibodies: serologic, physiologic, and clinical studies. In: Progress in Hematology. New York, NY: Grune & Stratton; 1964:222.

95. Colombani J, Colombani M, Dausset J. Two cases of neonatal thrombocytopenia due to maternal iso-immunization against leuko-platelet antigens. Vox Sang. 1968;14:137.

96. van Loghem JJ, Dorfmiester H, van der Hart M, et al. Serological and genetic studies on a platelet antigen (Zw). Vox Sang. 1959;4:161.

97. Mueller-Eckhardt C. Platelet allo- and autoantigens and their clinical implications. In: Nance ST, ed. Transfusion Medicine in the 1990s. Arlington, Va: American Association of Blood Banks; 1990.

98. Morrison SF, Mollison PL. Post-transfusion purpura. N Engl J Med. 1966;275:243.

99. Gockeman JP, Shulman NR. Isoantibody specificity in post-transfusion purpura. N Engl J Med. 1974;291:1163.

100. Abramason N, Eisenberg PD, Aster RH. Post-transfusion purpura: immunologic aspects and therapy. Blood. 1977;41:817.
101. Vaughan-Neil F, Ardeman S, Bevan G, et al. Post-transfusion purpura associated with an unusual platelet antibody (anti-PlB). Br Med J. 1975;1:436.
102. Ziegler Z, Murphy S, Gardner FH. Post-transfusion purpura: a heterogeneous syndrome. Blood. 1975;45:529.
103. Muller-Eckhardt C, Lechner K, Heinrich D, et al. Post-transfusion thrombocytopenic purpura: immunological and clinical studies in two cases and review of the literature. Blut. 1980;40:249.
104. Nichols RJ, Davies P, Kenwright NG. Thrombocytopenia and purpura after blood transfusion. Br Med J. 1970;2:581.
105. Dainer PM, Canada ED. Post-transfusion purpura and multiple transfusion. Br Med J. 1977;2:999.
106. Tanning E, Killman SA, Morling N, et al. Post-transfusion purpura (PTP) due to anti-Zwb-(PlA2): the significance of IgG antibodies in PTP. Br J Haematol. 1986;64:217.
107. Goldstein IM, Eyre HJ, Terasake PI, et al. Leukocyte transfusions: role of leukocyte alloantibodies in determining transfusion response. Transfusion. 1971;11:19.
108. Cimo PL, Aster RH. Post-transfusion purpura: successful treatment by exchange transfusion. N Engl J Med. 1972;287:290.
109. Harrington WJ. The clinical significance of antibodies for platelets. Paris: Communication of the Fifth International Congress of Hematology; 1954.
110. Aster RJ, Jandl JH. Platelet sequestration in man, II: immunological and clinical studies. J Clin Invest. 1964;43:856.
111. Allen JC, Kunkel HG. Antibodies to genetic types of gammaglobulin after multiple transfusion. Science. 1963;139:418.
112. Steinman ER, Fudenberg HH. Antibodies to gamma-globulin in infants and children exposed to isologous gamma-globulin. Pediatrics. 1965;35:229.
113. Allen JC, Kunkel HG. Antibodies against gamma-globulin after repeated blood transfusions in man. J Clin Invest. 1966;45:29.
114. Fudenberg HH, Steinman ER, Franklin EC, et al. Antigenicity of hereditary human gammaglobulin (Gm) factors: biological and chemical aspects. Cold Spring Harb Symp Quant Biol. 1964;29:463.
115. Barandun S, Kistler P, Jeunet F, et al. Intravenous administration of human gamma-globulin. Vox Sang. 1962;7:157.
116. Notes on epidemiology. Human immunoglobulin by the intravenous route. Br Med J. 1977;1:521.
117. Koisten J. Selective IgA deficiency in blood donors. Vox Sang. 1975;29:192.
118. Vyas GN, Perkins HA, Yang YM, et al. Healthy blood donors with selective absence of immunoglobulin A: prevention of anaphylactic transfusion reactions. J Lab Clin Med. 1975;85:838.
119. Holt PD, Tandy NP, Anstee DJ. Screening of blood donors for IgA deficiency: a study of the donor population of South-West England. J Clin Pathol. 1977;30:1007.
120. van Loghen JJ. Familial occurrence of selective IgA deficiency associated with antibody to IgA: evidence against a structural gene defect. Eur J Immunol. 1974;4:57.
121. Koistinen J, Sarna S. Immunological abnormalities in the sera of IgA-deficient blood donors. Vox Sang. 1975;29:203.
122. Vyas GN, Holmdahl L, Perkins HA, et al. Serological specificity of human anti-IgA and its significance in transfusion. Blood. 1969;34:573.
123. Vyas GN, Perkins HA, Fudenberg HH. Anaphylactoid transfusion reactions associated with anti-IgA. Lancet. 1968;2:312.
124. Schmidt AT, Taswell HF, Gleich GJ. Anaphylactic transfusion reactions associated with anti-IgA antibody. N Engl J Med. 1969;280:188.

125. Miller WV, Holland PV, Sugarbaker E, et al. Anaphylactic reactions to IgA: a difficult transfusion problem. Am J Clin Pathol. 1970;54:618.
126. Vyas GN. Antibodies to IgA causing anaphylactic reactions to small transfusions. American Association of Blood Banks Workshop on Transfusion Problems. Washington, DC: American Association of Blood Banks; 1970;2:21.
127. Bjerrum OJ, Jersild C. Class-specific IgA associated with severe anaphylactic transfusion reactions in a patient with pernicious anemia. Vox Sang. 1971;21:411.
128. Ropars C, Gerbal A, Poncey C, et al. Accident transfusionnel de type anaphylactique en rapport avec un anticorp anti-IgA. Rev Transfusion. 1971;14:401.
129. Leikola J, Vyas GN. Human antibodies to ruminant IgM concealing the absence of IgA in man. J Lab Clin Med. 1971;77:629.
130. Koistinen J, Leikola J. Weak anti-IgA antibodies with human specificity and nonhemolytic transfusion reactions. Vox Sang. 1977;32:77.
131. Rivat L, Rivat C, Parent P, et al. Accident survent aprés injection de g-globuline anti-Rh dû à la presence v'anticorps anti-g A. Presse Med. 1970;78:2072.
132. Mackenzie MR, Mackey G, Fudenberg HH. Antibodies to IgM in normal human sera. Nature. 1967;216:691.
133. Leikola J, Fudenberg HH, Vyas GN, et al. Isoantibodies to human IgM: serologic and immunologic investigations. J Immunol. 1971;106:1147.
134. Ropars C, Whylie S, Carton J, et al. Anticorps chez les polytransfuses direges contre certaines immunoglobulines IgM. Nouv Rev Fr Hematol. 1973;13:459.
135. Barton JC, Herrera GA, Galla JH, et al. Acute cryoglobulinemic renal failure after intravenous infusion of gammaglobulin. Am J Med. 1987;82:624.
136. Michel J, Sharoun R. Non-hemolytic adverse reaction after tranfusion of a blood unit containing penicillin. Br Med J. 1980;280:152.
137. Blumberg BS, Bernanke D, Allison AC. A human lipoprotein polymorphism. J Clin Invest. 1962;41:1936.
138. Hirshfeld J. The Ag system: present concepts and immunogenetic models. In: Peeters E, ed. Protides of the Biological Fluids. Oxford: Pergamon Press; 1972:156.
139. Butler R, Brunner E, Morganti G. Contributions to the inheritance of the Ag groups: a population genetic study. Vox Sang. 1974;26:485.

## Chapter 5

# Immunosuppression in Relation to Transfusion

It has been known for a number of years that the transfusion of blood products into recipients would precipitate modification in the immune response of those recipients to various immunologic challenges.[1-3] In particular, the observations of Opelz and Terasaki[4] introduced a new therapeutic modality, which resulted in great benefit to many patients, including the improved survival of renal allografts in patients receiving multiple transfusions of various blood components as compared to untransfused control subjects. Yet, even today, the mechanisms by which blood transfusion improves the host's immunologic tolerance to transplanted tissue are complex and not well understood.

Transfusion clearly has a number of demonstrable effects on certain aspects of immunologic function (Table 5-1). The definition of the factors that appear to benefit allograft survival, however, remains obscure. The issue to determine fully and resolve is whether or not the overall effect of transfusions may actually have some deleterious effects on the immune response considered as a whole. There are unquestionably some cases in which these negative effects may well obscure the more demonstrably beneficial ones. For example, it is possible that transfusions might improve immunologic tolerance not only toward tissue allografts but also, perhaps, toward certain types of neoplasms. Conversely, transfusions may alter unfavorably the immune response to certain types of infection.[3,4] Some recent evidence demonstrates that the progress of human immunodeficiency virus infection (HIV) from its clinically latent stage to fully developed acquired immunodeficiency syndrome (AIDS) is accelerated in patients who receive multiple transfusions of relatively large volumes of plasma or plasma-containing products as compared to those who receive a smaller number of RBC units.[5,6] This chapter will address these issues, and also some of the more significant observations relating to the practice of blood transfusion and modifications of the immune response. Particular emphasis will be given to clinical circumstances in which these effects may be variously classified as beneficial or potential deleterious.

**Table 5-1 Some Observed Effects on Immunologic Function Following Blood Transfusion in Patients With Chronic Renal Disease**

| Aspect Evaluated | Response After Transfusion |
|---|---|
| Mixed lymphocyte culture | Variable response |
| Response to soluble antigens or mitogens | Generally reduced |
| T-helper cells | Reduced in number |
| Natural killer cells | Reduced activity |
| Cell-mediated cytotoxicity | Variable response |

## Effects of Transfusion on Immune Function

### Renal Failure Patients

During the last decade, an extensive literature has developed from the original observations of Opelz and Terasaki[4] supporting the premise that preoperative blood transfusions have substantially improved the prospective survival of renal allografts in transplant recipients. Despite the more recent efforts of numerous investigators in the field, a complete understanding of the mechanisms involved is not yet available. The data presented in Table 5-1 provide a perspective of the observed effects of transfusion on immunologic function. The references cited represent a selected minority of the publications of principal investigators. The references are particularly pertinent to the area of renal allograft transplantation, and, while they do not show uniform agreement, they do concur that the overall effect is decidedly more beneficial than adverse.[7,21] For instance, the observed improvement in allograft survival, apparently induced by preoperative transfusion, is influenced by a number of factors.

#### *Type of Component Used*

There may be a relationship between the potential efficacy of preoperative transfusions in prolonging allograft survival and the probable WBC content of the blood component used.[22] Some reports suggest that even the use of frozen, deglycerolized, saline-suspended RBC concentrates exerts an observable positive effect on graft survival.[23,24] Others have found such transfusions to be either ineffective or of little benefit unless more than 4 transfusions are given.[25] Although the use of other leukocyte-poor preparations has shown much variance in their effect,[26] much more consistency has been found with the use of unwashed RBC concentrates, whole blood, or buffy coat preparations in the production of protective effects.

### *The Number of Transfusions Necessary*

There is still some question as to the optimal number of transfusions that are necessary to provide a beneficial result, although the benefits of preoperative transfusion in prospective renal allograft patients appear to far exceed the disadvantages in terms of graft survival. Claims have been made supporting the potential efficacy of even single component transfusions,[27,28] and a consensus suggests that a multiple transfusion protocol shows statistically significant benefits. The earlier conclusion that single transfusions may be comparably as effective as multiple ones has not been substantiated by experience.[29] It appears reasonable to conclude that several transfusions, perhaps as many as 5, are required for optimal effect but that no advantage can be demonstrated for greater than 5.[25]

### *Timing of the Transfusions*

There appears to be a relationship between the timing of preoperative transfusions in prospective allograft patients and the development of maximized beneficial effect. Transfusions administered more than 1 year or less than 10 days prior to grafting are likely to be of little benefit. On the other hand, best results seem to occur if transplantation is carried out between 1 and 6 months after the completion of the preoperative course of transfusions (ie, between 1 and 6 months after the last transfusion is administered).[30]

### *Donor-Specific Transfusions*

The use of donor-specific transfusion has been encouraging where it concerns the improvement of allograft survival rate in renal transplant patients. Donors are generally related and typically show 1 or 2 HLA antigen mismatches. Patients have been studied both with concomitant immunosuppressive therapy using prednisone and azathioprine during the period of transfusion or without such immunosuppression.[31] When the development of lymphocytotoxic antibodies, which might prejudice graft survival, appears significantly higher, more favorable results appear to be obtainable in those with concomitant immunosuppressive therapy.[32]

### *Lymphocytotoxicity Crossmatching and Graft Survival*

The issue of lymphocytotoxicity crossmatch compatibility between a prospective renal allograft recipient and the kidney donor is a complex one, but, depending on the nature of antibodies present in the recipient's plasma, it may be of considerable significance in predicting the possible outcome of transplantation. Table 5-2 lists the comparative significance of various types of histocompatibility antibody in prospective renal allograft recipients. In general, warm-reactive anti–T cell antibodies are deleterious and have been associated with hyperacute graft rejection. Warm anti–B cell antibodies may also be deleterious but show much more variation in effect. Cold antibodies (temperature optimum 4°C) directed against T cells are hard to evaluate in this context, whereas those of similar thermal range that are directed against B cells appear either to have no detectable effect or even to be beneficial. There is some evidence that patients who are negative by lymphocytotoxicity crossmatch at the time of transplantation have good allograft survival even if they had previously had a detectable T-cell antibody.[33] Thus, even though the recipient's immunologic memory may have been programmed by a previous immunizing event, and anamnestic stimulation of that memory by the allograft may be likely, a reasonable result may still be expected if the patient is antibody negative at the time of transplantation. This positive cause/effect relationship exists because concomitant immunosuppressive therapy predictably suppresses the expression of immunologic memory.

Voluminous data accumulated over the past decade collectively present a somewhat confused picture from which 3 conclusions may be drawn. First, in the majority of cases, there is little doubt that pretransplantation transfusion therapy results in the development of an immunologic tolerance of the donor by the recipient. Second, in some cases there appears to be a contrary effect: the stimulation of specific immunity to the donor. Third, a nonspecific, more-or-less general suppression of immune function is noted in still others. Pretransplantation transfusion can play a significant part in subsequent allograft survival and has a major role in the treatment of many patients with chronic renal failure, but the opposite effect may also result in some cases. In still other instances, a complex result may occur that involves the stimulation of some aspects of immunologic function and the suppression of others. The development of adverse immunologic consequences from pretransplantation transfusions, which occurs in some patients, must be considered as a very definite transfusion hazard.

### Patients With Coagulopathies

Various parameters have been studied in patients with major inherited coagulopathies (eg, hemophilia A, hemophilia B, and von Willebrand's disease), that measure different aspects of the immune response when treated with human plasma or human plasma derivatives. Such studies have included response to mixed lymphocyte culture,[34] in vitro response to soluble antigens or mitogens,[35-40] the numbers of T-helper

**Table 5-2** Comparative Significance of Various Histocompatibility Antibodies in Relation to Renal Allografts

| Classification | Antibody Type | Probable Effect on Allograft |
| --- | --- | --- |
| I | Anti-T cell antibodies | |
| | Warm reacting (37°C) | Deleterious |
| | Cold reacting (4°C) | Uncertain (rare) |
| II | Anti-B cell antibodies | |
| | Warm reacting (37°C) | Neutral or harmful |
| | Cold reacting (4°C) | Neutral or beneficial |

compared with suppressor cells,[37,41-45] monocyte function,[46] and the activity of natural killer cells[47-49] in general. The recorded responses to the use of plasma products in these patients with coagulopathies have been negative on balance. Many patients have shown reduced responses in mixed lymphocyte culture and in the in vitro response of their cells to stimulation by soluble antigens or mitogens, whereas many others have shown decreased numbers of T-helper cells with increased numbers or activity of suppressor cells.[50] Other reports have suggested that dysfunction (pre-existing immunosuppression) in such patients, complicated by HIV-1 infection, may be expected to result in the progression of this disease to the development of full-blown AIDS. Many cases exhibit immune suppression of varying degrees, measured by these criteria. Thus, the overall significance of this immunosuppression may be difficult to evaluate. It may also be true that the development of objective criteria for immunosuppression can result in some cases from otherwise occult HIV-1 infection prior to the development of a positive serologic result. Other viruses may also be responsible for these changes. Fortunately, significant progress is being made in the development of coagulation factor concentrates that are either free from or at greatly reduced risk for transfusion-transmissible viruses.[51]

### Patients With Hemoglobinopathies

Another group of patients frequently subjected to repeated transfusion therapy are those suffering from inherited hemoglobinopathies, in particular thalassemia and sickle cell anemia. In contrast to patients with coagulopathies whose requirements are for plasma or plasma derivatives, patients with hemoglobinopathy require frequent transfusion with RBCs or washed RBCs to maintain an acceptable hemoglobin level. Although it can be shown that such patients do exhibit definable changes in immune function, these changes are generally less pronounced and severe than those encountered in hemophiliacs. This finding raises a number of questions about the difference between these 2 groups (those receiving plasma derivatives and those receiving essentially RBC concentrates).

First, 1 difference is obvious: the infusion of coagulation factor concentrates (made from pooled human plasma prior to the availability of heat-inactivated material, monoclonal material, or otherwise refined and relatively virus-free concentrates) carried with it a greatly increased risk of viral transmission. In particular this included HIV-1 and the various viruses associated with transfusion hepatitis. A single dose of such a concentrate made in this way and otherwise unmodified carries many times the risk of viral transmission compared to single-donor units of RBCs, with or without plasma. This risk was clearly reflected in the much lower incidence of HIV-1 infections in patients with hemoglobinopathies who were receiving frequent RBC transfusions as compared to those with coagulopathies who were receiving frequent infusions of pooled coagulation factor concentrates.[52-54]

Another potential contributory factor in the development of variable immunosuppression is the iron overload seen regularly in these patients, both as a result of continued hemolysis and of transfusion.[53,54] Iron overload has been implicated as the possible cause of neutrophil phagocytic dysfunction in renal failure patients who are undergoing chronic hemodialysis.[55] This has not been convincingly demonstrated, however, in multiply transfused patients with hemoglobinopathies. Claims that macrophage system functions are impaired in such multiply transfused individuals have also been offset by the contrary findings of others.[56,57] It cannot be shown convincingly that such patients are at greater overall risk for bacterial and other infections than the general population.

## Other Conditions

A number of observations pose considerable interest with relation to alterations in the immune response in certain groups of patients who may be subject to intense transfusion therapy using a variety of blood components for a relatively short period. These have included cardiac surgical patients,[58] newborns who have received exchange transfusion,[59,61] and some patients with recurrent gastrointestinal inflammatory disease, notably regional ileitis and ulcerative colitis.[60] Patients who had received exchange transfusions of whole blood from homologous donors as newborns still showed some abnormalities of immune function for up to 20 years after the event. In particular, this dysfunction was manifested by a diminished response in the mixed lymphocyte culture test. Patients with recurrent inflammatory bowel disease receiving multiple transfusions of RBCs showed significant reduction in total numbers of circulating lymphocytes. They also showed alterations in reactivity to skin tests for up to 18 months after the last transfusion.[62] There was a positive correlation between the degree of immunologic abnormality and the number of units transfused, particularly in patients undergoing resective surgery with copious perioperative transfusion. In these groups of patients, such complicating and possibly confusing factors as viral infection, iron overload, or the concomitant effects of major trauma could be excluded, leading to the conclusion that the acquisition of varying degrees of immune deficiency correlated closely with blood transfusion.

## Effects of Plasma Transfusion on the Course of HIV Infection

Early cases of AIDS associated with blood transfusion were reported occurring in patients who had received massive blood transfusion, including the use of plasma-rich components. In HIV infections, viral replication and disease progression are enhanced by factors known to bring about immunologic suppression, such as the therapeutic use of steroids.[63] Some early observations suggested that the type of blood component transfused to a patient infected with HIV had little or no influence on the rate at which this condition progressed from a latent state to either AIDS-related complex (ARC) or to full-blown AIDS.[64]

George and Morello[2] reported statistical studies of the progress of HIV infection in patients transfused with a variety of blood components. Their conclusions are significant. Whereas RBC transfusions accounted for 66% of surviving HIV-infected patients, only 32% of the cases (9 of 28) that progressed to AIDS occurred among regular recipients of RBC transfusions, as distinct from those receiving plasma-rich products.[65] Moreover, it has been shown that there is a positive correlation between the dosage of plasma received by an HIV-infected patient and progression to AIDS, as compared to those infected but remaining asymptomatic despite some degree of further transfusion.[2] In the reported study, patients receiving a median dosage of approximately 450 mL of plasma have remained asymptomatic, whereas, in those who progressed to the development of AIDS, the median dosage of plasma was 1500 mL.

Progression of asymptomatic HIV infection to AIDS is significantly less frequent in patients who receive washed or frozen, deglycerolized saline-suspended RBC concentrates as distinct from those who receive plasma-rich components. While components that are leukocyte-poor can be expected to deliver small numbers of virus-laden WBCs to the recipient, they are equally poor or even totally deficient in plasma. Possibly, they may therefore be as deficient in immunosuppressive plasma constituents.[66-68] It has also been observed that children receiving blood transfusions for the treatment of malaria show a substantially increased risk of acquiring HIV infection than can be accounted for by the plain risk of exposure.[69]

Based on careful statistical analysis of detailed reports showing the progression of HIV infection to ARC or AIDS in association with blood transfusions, the available evidence indicates that the infection is adversely affected by multiple transfusion of plasma-rich products and that it is less likely to occur, other things being equal, in recipients of RBC transfusions only, particularly if these are washed or frozen and deglycerolized. It will be interesting to see whether corresponding figures of patients treated with RBC transfusions in which the RBC concentrates were rendered leukocyte-poor by selective leukocyte filtration rather than washing will show any difference from the observed figures from transfusion of washed RBCs.

## Blood Transfusion and Cancer

In 1982, Burrows and Tartter[70] reported an observed adverse effect of perioperative blood transfusions on the recurrence of chronic anorectal cancer: that they can in fact be shown to have a statistically significant, deleterious effect on cancer recurrence. Later studies[71-73] confirmed their impression. Since these earlier observations, some reports have apparently corroborated these impressions,[74-76] whereas others have found no adverse correlation between transfusion and cancer recurrence.[77-79] Various other studies (some involving multiple cases and others involving only few or single cases but with a diverse array of tumors including lung, breast, kidney, prostate, stomach, head and neck cancer, and soft tissue sarcoma) tend to confirm the impression that blood transfusions affect the rate of recurrence of most of these malignancies adversely.[80-93] An exception is breast cancer, which did not appear to show this correlation.[92-94] Blumberg et al[95] found that transfusion of multiple units of whole blood, as distinct from RBC concentrates, is associated with a significantly higher recurrence rate and a poorer prognosis for many patients with cancer. They speculate that whole blood may contain a distinctly greater quantity of leukocyte debris and other material, particulate and solubilized, that might be capable of bringing about adverse suppression of immune function. Certainly, their studies demonstrate that the situation concerning cancer recurrence is much more favorable in patients who receive only a single unit of RBCs or of whole blood than in those receiving multiple whole blood transfusions. The difference is dramatically emphasized in the significantly worsened prognosis of patients who receive only a single unit of whole blood, compared to those receiving a single unit of RBCs.[95]

Not too surprisingly, of the various components used, whole blood appears to produce the most favorable results on cadaveric renal allograft survival. This may be due specifically to its high content of WBC remnants and their associated histocompatibility antigens, together with solubilized antigenic material. Less favorable results are seen with unwashed

RBC concentrates and relatively poor results with washed or frozen, deglycerolized RBCs. The relative importance of the various constituents (plasma constituents, cellular debris, solubilized antigens, etc) in producing immunologic tolerance for allografted material or cancer cells in the recipient or host is still controversial.

Intravenous administration of high-dose immunoglobulin preparations appears to modify the immune response.[96-98] Beneficial effects of such administration on pneumonia associated with cytomegalovirus have been attributed to a nonspecific immunosuppressive effect produced by the preparation.[99] Recently, a number of studies have shown that Class I histocompatibility antigens, which accumulate abundantly in stored human blood, are highly efficient in inhibiting alloreactive cytotoxic T cells.[100] It has also been shown that soluble Class I histocompatibility antigens are present in significant amounts in human plasma derivatives, such as coagulation factor concentrates, and that a positive correlation exists between the immunosuppressive qualities of such concentrates and the content of these soluble antigens.[101] Soluble plasma antigens, serum, and some constituents of anticoagulant solutions, such as adenine and even sodium citrate, may adversely affect the mixed lymphocyte culture response.[102,103]

## Conclusion

The whole relationship between transfusion of blood components and derivatives and modification or suppression of the immune response is complex. Furthermore, its clinical relevance is difficult to evaluate. There is no doubt as to the efficacy of the transfusion of certain blood components on the survival of renal allografts. However, more recent observations of this phenomenon in current practice indicate a decrease in effectiveness.[104,105] Techniques for the preparation of RBC components involving more complete expression of plasma and virtually the complete removal of WBC constituents and the material by improved filtration techniques may well account for this change. Certainly, a more detailed study on the mechanisms involved and the application of the results of such studies to the preparation of "cleaner" blood components is going to be necessary.[106]

At the risk of being called heretical, I would suggest that there is still a definite place for washed RBC components and for the use of frozen, deglycerolized saline-suspended RBCs in certain selected clinical circumstances. By eliminating both plasma and leukocyte-related material, including most of the solubilized histocompatibility antigens, blood transfusion may yet be rendered safer in patients with certain kinds of cancers or for those suffering from certain viral infections (eg, HIV) whose biologic behavior is only imperfectly appreciated.

## References

1. Anstall HB. Transfusion therapy in special clinical situations. In: Anstall HB, Urie PM. A Manual of Hemotherapy. New York, NY: John Wiley and Sons; 1986:267.
2. George CD, Morello PJ. Immunologic effects of blood transfusion upon renal transplantation, tumor operations, and bacterial infection. Am J Surg. 1986;152:329.
3. Blumberg N, Heal JM. Perioperative blood transfusion and solid tumor recurrence. Blood Rev. 1987;1:219.
4. Opelz G, Terasaki PI. Improvement of kidney graft survival with increased numbers of blood transfusions. N Engl J Med. 1978;299:799.
5. Blumberg N, Heal JM. Transfusion and recipient immune function. Pathol Lab Med. 1989;113:246.
6. Wachter JF, Fuchs D, Hausman A, et al. Are conditions linked with T-cell stimulation necessary for progressive HTLD III infections? Lancet. 1986;1:97.
7. Salvatiera O, Vincent FA, Amend W, et al. Deliberate donor-specific blood transfusion prior to living-related renal transplantation. Ann Surg. 1980;192:543.
8. Leivestad T, Thorsby E. Effects of HLA-haploidentical blood transfusions on donor-specific immune responsiveness. Transplantation. 1984;37:175.
9. Cheigh JS, Suthanthiran M, Kaplan M, et al. Induction of immune alterations and successful renal transplantation: a simplified method of donor-specific blood transfusion. Transplantation. 1984;38:501.
10. Sanfilipo F, Crawford J, Ness G, et al. Influence of donor-specific blood transfusions on host cellular immune responsiveness. Transplant Proc. 1986;18:692.
11. Keown P, Descamps B. Suppression de la reaction lymphocytaire mixte par les globules rouges autologues leazt leurs constituants. C R Acta Sci. 1978;287:749.
12. Fehrman I, Ringden O. Lymphocytes from multitransfused uremic patients have poor MLC reactivity. Tissue Antigens. 1981;17:386.
13. Kerman RH, Agostino G, van Burren CT, et al. Effect of blood transfusion on graft survival and immune responsiveness. Transplant Proc. 1983;15:1005.
14. Klatzmann D, Gluckman JG, Chapuis F, et al. Suppression of lymphocyte reactivity by blood transfusion in uremic patients. Transplantation. 1984;38:232.
15. Tait BD, d'Appice AJ, Morrow L, et al. Changes in suppressor-cell activity in renal dialysis patients after blood transfusion. Transplant Proc. 1984;16:995.
16. Roy R, Lachance JG, Noel R, et al. Improved renal allograft function and survival following nonspecific blood transfusions. Transplantation. 1986;41:640.
17. Schot JDL, Schurmann RKB. Blood transfusion suppresses cutaneous cell-mediated immunity. Clin Exp Immunol. 1986;65:336.
18. Mohanakumar T, Ellis TM, Mendez-Picon G, et al. Monitoring human T-cell subpopulations, effects of immunosuppressive therapy and blood transfusion on OKT4+/OKT8+ ratios. Transplant Proc. 1983;15:1978.
19. Nanishi F, Inenaga T, Omoyama K, et al. Immune alterations in hemodialyzed patients, I: effect of blood transfusion on T-lymphocyte subpopulations in hemodialyzed patients. J Clin Lab Immunol. 1986;19:167.
20. Matsumoto T, Sakagami K, Tsuboi K, et al. Possible mechanism of donor-specific blood transfusions in prolongation of graft survival. Transplant Proc. 1985;17:2401.
21. Ford CD, Warnick CT, Sheets S, et al. Blood transfusions or actual killer cell activity. Transplant Proc. 1987;19:1456.
22. Lasitey LC. Transfusion in chronic renal disease. In: Umas J, Silvergleid AJ, eds. Transfusion for the Patient with Selected Clinical Problems. Arlington, Va: American Association of Blood Banks; 1982.
23. Valtis JC, Kennedy AC. The cause and prevention of defective function of stirred red blood cells after transfusion. Glasgow Med J. 1953;34:552.

24. Ciciarelli JD, Terasaki P. Immunological aspects of HLA cross-matching and transfusion in kidney transplantation. In: Garratty G, ed. Blood Group Antigens and Disease: A Technical Workshop. Arlington, Va: American Association of Blood Banks; 1983.

25. Opelz G, Terasaki PI. International study of histocompatibility in renal transplantation. Transplantation. 1982;33:87.

26. Vincenti F, Duca RM, Amend W, et al. Immunological factors determining the survival of cadaveric kidney transplants. N Engl J Med. 1978;299:293.

27. Werner-Faure C, Jeannet M, Harder F, et al. Blood transfusions, cytotoxic antibodies, and kidney graft survival. Transplantation. 1979;28:343.

28. Corry RJ, West JC, Hunsicker LC, et al. Effect of timing of administration and quantity of blood transfusions on cadaveric renal transplant survival. Transplantation. 1980;30:425.

29. Sirach G, Merculali F, Salamongna M, et al. Evaluation of the blood transfusion policy of north Italy transplantation program. Transplantation. 1981;31:388.

30. Manducci PM, Paretti SI, Ruggeri CM, et al. 1-Deamino-8-d-arginine vasopressin: a new pharmacological approach to the management of hemophilia A and von Willebrand's disease. Lancet. 1977;1:669.

31. Fuller TC, Delmonico FL, Cosmi AB, et al. Effect of various types of red blood cell transfusions on HLA alloimmunization and renal allograft survival. Transplant Proc. 1977;9:117.

32. Ciciarelli JL, Chia V, Terasaki PI, et al. Human IgM anti-IgM cytotoxin of B lymphocytes. Tissue Antigens. 1980;15:275.

33. Cardella CJ, Falk JA. Graft outcome in patients with antibodies reactive with donor T and B cells. Transplant Rev. 1983;15:114.

34. Gjerset GF, Martin PJ, Counts RB, et al. Immunological status of hemophilia patients treated with cryoprecipitate or lyophilized concentrate. Blood. 1984;64:715.

35. Bretter DB, Forsberg AD, Brewster F, et al. Delayed cutaneous hypersensitivity reaction in hemophiliac subjects treated with Octor concentrate. Am J Med. 1986;81:607.

36. Kekow J, Plendl H, Gross WL, et al. Abnormal B ison cell response to T-cell-independent polyclonal b-cell activities in hemophilia A. Clin Exp Immunol. 1986;64:376.

37. Sharp RA, Moreley SM, Beck JS, et al. Unresponsiveness to skin testing with bacterial antigens in patients with hemophilia A not apparently infected with human immunodeficiency virus (HIV). J Clin Pathol. 1987;40:849.

38. Matheson DS, Green BJ, Fritzler MJ, et al. Humoral immune response in patients with hemophilia. Clin Immunol Immunopathol. 1987;4:41.

39. Brettler DB, Brewster F, Levine PH, et al. Immunologic aberrations, HIV seropositivity and seroconversion rates in patients with hemophilia B. Blood. 1987;70:276.

40. Freedman J, Mazaheri R, Read S, et al. Humoral and cellular immune abnormalities in adult hemophiliacs followed over a two-year period. Diagn Clin Immunol. 1987;5:30.

41. Moffat EH, Bloom AL, Jones J, et al. A study of cell-mediated and humoral immunity in hemophilia and related disorders. Br J Haematol. 1985;61:157.

42. Wearne A, Joshua DE, Rickard KA, et al. Abnormal T-cell subpopulations in hemophilic patients recieving factor VIII caps concentrates from voluntary donors. Aust N Z J Med. 1984;14:149.

43. Pollack S, Atias D, Yoffe G, et al. Impaired immune function in hemophilia patients treated exclusively with cryoprecipitate: relation to duration of treatment. Am J Hematol. 1985;20:1.

44. Smolen S, Bettelheim P, Koller U, et al. Deficiency of the autologous mixed lymphocyte reaction in patients with classic hemophilia treated with commercial factor VIII concentrates. J Clin Invest. 1975;75:1828.

45. Jason J, Hilgartner M, Holman RC, et al. Immune status of blood product recipients. JAMA. 1985;253:1140.
46. Eible MM, Ahmad R, Wolf HM, et al. A component of factor VIIA preparations which can be separated from factor VIII activity that modulates human monocyte function. Blood. 1987;69:1153.
47. Goicoa MA, Estevez ME, Ballart IJ, et al. Impairment of natural (NK) killer function in carriers and patients with thalassemia major. Nouv Rev Fr Hematol. 1986;28:75.
48. Kaplan JS, Sarnaik SL, Levy J. Transfusion-induced immunologic abnormalities not related to AIDS virus. N Engl J Med. 1985;213:1227.
49. Choremia H, Sidiri E, Psarra K, et al. Immune status of Greek patients with beta-thalassemia major negative for anti-HIV. Blut. 1987;54:267.
50. Kaplan J, Sarnaik S, Gitlin J, et al. Diminished helper/suppressor lymphocyte ratios and natural killer activity in recipients of repeated blood transfusions. Blood. 1984;64:308.
51. Sullivan JL, Brewster FE, Brettler DB, et al. Hemophiliac immunodefiency: influence of exposure to factor VIII concentrate, LAV/HTLV-III and herpesviruses. J Pediatr. 1986;108:504.
52. Wang W, Herrod H, Presbury G, et al. Lymphocyte phenotype and function in chronically transfused children with sickle-cell disease. Am J Hematol. 1985;20:31.
53. DeMartino M, Rossi ME, Muccioli ALT, et al. Altered T-cell subsets and function in polytransfused beta-thalassemia patients: correlation with sex and age at first transfusion. Vox Sang. 1985;48:296.
54. Pardalos G, Kanakoudi-Tsakalidis F, Malaka-Zafiriu M, et al. Iron-related disturbances of cell-mediated immunity in multitransfused children with thalassemia major. Clin Exp Immunol. 1987;68:138.
55. Waterlot Y, Cantinieaux B, Hariga-Muller C. Impaired phagocytic activities of neutrophils in patients receiving hemodialysis. Br J Med. 1985;291:501.
56. Szymanski IO, Elfath MD, Huff SR. The site of destruction of stored nonviable red blood cells (RBC), abstracted. Clin Res. 1987;35:43.
57. Dimitriou P, Giannouris G, Nicolaidou P, et al. RES phagocytosis in children with homozygous beta-thalassemia major in relation to blood transfusion. Scand J Hematol. 1986;37:41.
58. Fernandez LA, MacSween JM, You CK, et al. Study of immunological changes after blood transfusion, abstracted. Blood. 1985;66:276.
59. Back L, Scott JS, Pepper M, et al. The effect of neonatal exchange and later blood transfusion on lymphocyte cultures. Am J Reprod Immunol. 1981;1:224.
60. Pahwa S, Sia C, Harp R, et al. Lymphocyte subpopulations in high-risk infants: influence of age and blood transfusion. Pediatrics. 1985;76:914.
61. Romano M, El Marsafy A, Marseglia GL, et al. Increased percentage of activated Ia+T-lymphocytes in the peripheral blood of neonates following exchange blood transfusion. Clin Immunol Immunopathol. 1987;43:301.
62. Tartte PI, Heimann TN, Aufses AI, et al. Blood transfusion, skin test reactivity, and lymphocytes in inflammatory bowel disease. Am J Surg. 1986;151:358.
63. Watcher J, Fuchs D, Hausen A, et al. Are conditions linked with T-cell stimulation necessary for HTLV-III in section? Lancet. 1986;1:197.
64. Peterman TA, Jaffe JW, Seorino PM, et al. Transfusion-associated AIDS in the United States. JAMA. 1985;254:2913.
65. Donegan E, Perkins H, Byas G, et al. Mortality of the recipients of blood in the transfusion safety study. Blood. 1986;68(suppl):296a.
66. Edelbaum DMN. No AIDS among patients on dialysis? N Engl J Med. 1986;314:187.
67. Prinseau J, Baglin A, Fruchart MF, et al. Survue d'un SIDA chez une hemodialysee clinique contaminee lors d'un transfusion sanguine. Sen Hosp Paris. 1988;64:925.

68. DeMartino M, Quarta G, Melpigniao A, et al. Antibodies to HTLV-III and the lymphadenopathy syndrome in multitransfused beta-thalassemia patients. Vox Sang. 1986;50:192.

69. Greenberg AE, Nguy-Dinh P, Mann JM. The association between malaria, blood transfusions, and HIV seropositivity in a pediatric population in Kinshasha, Zaire. JAMA. 1988;259:545.

70. Burrows L, Tartter P. Effect of blood transfusions on colonic malignance. Lancet. 1982;2:662.

71. Agarwal M, Blumberg N. Colon cancer patients transfused perioperatively have an increased incidence of recurrence. Transfusion. 1983;23:421.

72. Blumberg N, Agarwal M, Chuang C. Relation between recurrence of cancer of the colon and blood transfusion. Br Med J. 1985;290:1037.

73. Foster RS, Costanza MC, Foster JC, et al. Adverse relationship between blood transfusions and survival after colectomy for colon cancer. Cancer. 1985;5:1195.

74. Corman J, Arnoux R, Peloquin A, et al. Blood transfusions and survival after colectomy for colorectal cancer. Can J Surg. 1986;29:325.

75. Parrott NR, Lemnard LWJ, Taylor RMR, et al. Effect of preoperative blood transfusion on recurrence of colorectal cancer. Br J Surg. 1986;73:970.

76. Voogt TJ, van der Velde CJH, Brand A, et al. Perioperative blood transfusion and cancer prognosis. Cancer. 1987;59:836.

77. Weiden PL, Bean MA, Schulz P. Perioperative blood transfusion does not increase the risk of colorectal cancer recurrence. Cancer. 1987;60:670.

78. Frankis PD, McNee RK, Alley PG, et al. Relation between cancer of the colon and blood transfusion. Br Med J. 1985;290:1827.

79. Blair SD, Janvrin SB. Relation between cancer of the colon and blood transfusion. Br Med J. 1985;290:1516.

80. Francis DM, Judson RI. Blood transfusion and recurrence of cancer of the colon and rectal. Br J Surg. 1987;74:26.

81. Creasey TS, Veitch PS, Bell PB, et al. Relation between perioperative blood transfusion and recurrence of carcinoma of the sigmoid colon following potentially curative surgery. Ann R Coll Surg Engl. 1987;69:100.

82. Ota D, Alvarez L, Lichtiger B, et al. Postoperative blood transfusions in patients with colon carcinoma. Transfusion. 1985;25:392.

83. Nathanson SD, Tilley BC, Schulz L, et al. Perioperative allogenic blood transfusions: survival in patients with resected carcinomas of the colon and rectum. Arch Surg. 1985;120:734.

84. Tarter PI, Burrows L, Kirschner P. Perioperative blood transfusion adversely affects prognosis after resection of state I (subset NO) non–oat cell lung cancer. J Thorac Cardiovasc Surg. 1984;88:659.

85. Hyman NH, Foster RS, Demeules JE, et al. Blood transfusions and survival after lung cancer resection. Am J Surg. 1985;149:502.

86. Pastorino U, Valente M, Cataldo I, et al. Perioperative blood transfusions and prognosis of resected stage Ia lung cancer. Eur J Cancer Clin. Oncol. 1986;22:1378.

87. Nowak MM, Ponsky JL. Blood transfusion and disease-free survival in carcinoma of the breast. Surg Oncol. 1984;27:124.

88. Tarter PI, Burrows L, Papatestas AE, et al. Perioperative blood transfusion has prognostic significance for breast cancer. Surgery. 1985;97:225.

89. Moffat LE, Sunderland GT, Lamont D. Blood transfusion and survival following nephrectomy for carcinoma of the kidney. Br J Urol. 1987;60:316.

90. Manyonda IT, Shaw DE, Foulkes A, et al. Renal cell carcinoma: blood transfusions and survival. Br Med J. 1986;293:537.

91. Mikulin T, Powell CS, Urwin GH, et al. Relation between blood transfusion and survival in renal adenocarcinoma. Br J Surg. 1986;73:1036.

92. Rosenberg SA, Seippo CA, White DE, et al. Perioperative blood transfusions are associated with increased rates of recurrence and decreased survival in patients with high-grade soft tissue sarcomas of the extremities. J Clin Oncol. 1985;3:698.
93. Kaneda M, Horini T, Ninomiya M, et al. Adverse effect of blood transfusions on survival of patients with gastric carcinoma. Transfusion. 1987;27:375.
94. Johnson JT, Taylor FH, Thearle PB. Blood transfusion and outcome in stage III head and neck carcinoma. Arch Otolaryngol Head Neck Surg. 1987;113:307.
95. Blumberg N, Agarwal M, Chang C. A poor association between survival time and transfusion in patients with cervical cancer. Yale J Biol Med. 1988;61:493-500.
96. Dalrymple JC, Monaghan JM. Recurrent carcinoma of the vulva relationship with operative blood transfusion. J Obstet Gynecol. 1988;7:65.
97. Heal JM, Chang C, Blumberg N. Preoperative blood transfusions in prostate carcinoma: recurrence and survival. Am J Surg. 1988;156:374.
98. Blumberg N, Heal JM, Murphy P, et al. The association between number of red cell transfusions and cancer recurrence suggests a dose-response relationship. Blood. 1986;68(suppl 1):29.
99. Blumberg N, Heal JM, Murphy P, et al. Further evidence supporting a cause and effect relationship between blood transfusion and earlier cancer recurrence. Ann Surg. 1988;207:410.
100. Riggio RR, Cheigh JS, Stenzel KH, et al. Kidney transplant: use of gamma globulin as an immunosuppressive agent. N Y State J Med. 1980;80:15.
101. England D, Waner JL, Kapoor N, et al. Effect of intravenous immune globulin on natural killer cell activity: possible associations with autoimmune neutropenia and idiopathic thrombocytopenia. J Pediatr. 1986;108:77.
102. Lee CA, Kernoff PBA, Karayiannia P, et al. Abnormal T-lymphocyte subset in hemophilia: relation to HLA proteins in plasma products. N Engl J Med. 1984;310:1058.
103. Vliet W, Dock N, Davey FR, et al. Factors in the liquid portion of stored blood inhibit the proliferation response in mixed lymphocyte culture. Transfusion. 1987;27:508A.
104. McDonald C, Jackson V, Kilpatrick DC, et al. A diffusable factor in Scottish coagulation factor concentrates can inhibit lymphocyte transformation in vitro. Vox Sang. 1985;49:187.
105. Time to abandon pretransplant blood transfusion? Lancet. 1988;1:567.
106. Blumberg N, Heal JM. Renal allograft survival in transfused and nontransfused patients. Lancet. 1988;1:946.

# CHAPTER 6

# NONIMMUNOLOGIC HAZARDS OF BLOOD TRANSFUSION

## PHYSICAL AND MECHANICAL HAZARDS

### Circulatory Hypervolemia

The administration of large quantities of blood or blood products can occasionally result in circulatory overload and congestion. This reaction may be severe enough to precipitate congestive cardiac failure or even death. Unless patients have experienced pre-existing cardiopulmonary disease, circulatory overload is generally associated with rapid infusion of large volumes of blood products, usually whole blood. Congestion may develop rapidly in those patients who show evidence of anxiety and restlessness, tachycardia, and varying degrees of dyspnea and cyanosis. In patients with either pre-existing cardiopulmonary disease or chronic anemia, even relatively small volumes of blood transfusion, especially when rapidly infused, can precipitate circulatory overload or congestive cardiac failure. In such cases, congestive failure may develop rapidly, with acute pulmonary edema being a possible result. In other cases, a more gradual onset of failure may be observed. Since blood transfusion should always be regarded as a hazardous procedure, meticulous monitoring and supervision must be required for those patients in these categories, particularly when several units of RBCs are to be administered.

As a general rule, patients with chronic anemia should not be transfused unless they are symptomatic and show evidence of either cardiovascular decompensation (high-output failure) or organ ischemia (myocardial, cerebrovascular). When there are no apparent symptoms and signs indicating either an ischemic threat to major organs or overt evidence of cardiovascular decompensation, but the hematocrit is greater than 24% and the hemoglobin is greater than 8 g/dL, patients should probably not be transfused with RBC concentrates. However, transfusion may be permissible in some patients with slightly higher hematocrits, particularly those in the middle-age to elderly category who reside at higher altitudes. A good rule of thumb is to avoid transfusion unless patients are symptomatic, especially when the hematocrit is greater than 24% and the hemoglobin is greater than 8 g/dL.

The risk of precipitating dangerous circulatory overload is highest in patients who show signs of cardiovascular decompensation prior to transfusion. In these cases, which are often associated with severe chronic anemia, administration of RBCs will generally foster significant and rapid improvement. These same patients may also be highly sensitive to sudden increases in total blood volume. Although the hematocrit may be greatly reduced, the total circulating volume is not; thus, the addition of any liquid component can be expected to elevate further and expand the total volume, at least transiently. Active treatment of incipient or actual congestive failure should be established whenever possible before undertaking the transfusion. Digitalis, diuretics, and oxygen should be used as necessary to optimize the patient's cardiovascular condition. If there is any evidence initially of increased central venous pressure, it is advisable to monitor either that pressure or pulmonary artery pressure. After the patient has been placed in a sitting position, the rate of transfusion should be carefully monitored. A slow rate of infusion is desirable and imperative when symptoms and signs of cardiovascular decompensation are present. If signs of circulatory overload do develop, the transfusion should be interrupted, and oxygen and diuretics should be administered. In urgent cases, therapeutic phlebotomy may be undertaken and is generally highly effective in controlling an emergency situation.[1]

## Microaggregate Infusion

During the course of storage, microaggregates (composed of platelets, leukocytes, and leukocyte fragments) and small amounts of fibrin gradually form, reaching their peak after some 14 days of shelf life, at which point they show a fairly wide range of particle size, varying from 10 to 200 μm in diameter. Microaggregates that develop in stored blood products can be quantitated approximately either by measuring the pressure required to permit a constant rate of flow of blood through a barrier-screen type of microaggregate filter (a measurement defined as "screen filtration pressure" [SFP]) or by noting the incremental weight of a filter observed after passing a defined volume of blood through it.[2,3] It can be shown that microaggregate formation probably begins within 24 hours in acid citrate dextrose (ACD) and citrate phosphate dextrose (CPD), and even earlier in heparin, using a variety of techniques and media, including scanning electron microscopy of defibrinated plasma and platelet-enriched serum, as well as whole blood and RBCs. Notable increases in SFP develop between 5 to 14 days and appear to correlate with fibrin formation.[3,4] During this period, the observed increase in SFP is generally higher in CPD-stored components than in those in which the anticoagulant is ACD.[5] Studies indicate that, while platelet-derived fibrin (rather than plasma-derived material) is responsible for the increase in SFP, fibrin formation appears to be the principal cause of it.[3] Some studies also indicate that some of the larger microaggregates disintegrate with prolonged storage (greater than 2 weeks).[3,6]

In the early to mid-1970s, it was strongly believed that acute respiratory distress, occurring in massively transfused trauma patients and combat casualties, resulted from microembolization of the pulmonary capillary bed by microaggregates accumulating in stored blood. This conclusion appeared to be supported by experiments in dogs. When transfused with blood stored over various periods of time, these dogs developed respiratory distress and increased pulmonary venous pressure. Lesions discovered on the dogs during autopsy were believed to have resulted from release of lysosomal contents from disintegrating microaggregates.[7,11] Further experience with battle casualties suggested, however, that thoracic injuries, particularly when complicated with infection, more frequently caused pulmonary insufficiency and respiratory distress than embolization by microaggregates.[12,13] Also, other experiments involving the massive transfusion of baboons supported these clinical observations.[14] These particular experiments, which created hypovolemic shock by inducing partial exsanguination via the passage of stored blood containing microaggregates through a standard (170 μm) blood filter, did not result in pulmonary insufficiency.

The significance of microaggregates in transfusion remains somewhat controversial. Leukocyte-specific filtration of blood components has largely replaced the previous routine use of microaggregate filters of 25 to 40 μm pore-size. The present clinical position, which seems tenable, calls for restricting the use of microaggregate filters to those high-volume transfusions cases where trauma and/or surgery involving thoracic injury or preexisting cardiopulmonary disease is required. In these exceptional cases, the use of microaggregate filtration is probably warranted.

## Air Embolism

The use of collapsible blood containers for the collection, storage, and administration of blood components has virtually eliminated venous air embolism as a transfusion hazard. These new containers are devoid of air and can be easily compressed either manually or by the use of externally applied inflatable devices.

Venous air embolism was occasionally observed when rigid glass bottles were used as blood containers. Operating from this old format, an external air vent was required to permit the free infusion of blood, which was then replaced in the container by air as it flowed into the patient. In emergent situations, the infusion rate could be greatly increased by attaching a syringe device to the vent and then manually pumping air into the container. This process caused the blood to expel at a higher rate. The significant risk of air embolism from various amounts of air that this procedure generated sometimes produced fatal consequences. Estimates of the volume of air necessary to produce a fatal result range from 10 to 200 mL.[15-17]

Some risks of venous air embolism also occurred with early cell separator devices. Modern refinements, however, have virtually eliminated air embolism as a hazard. Examples of these refinements are the incorporation of an air-bubble trap on the return line and pressure-sensitive censors that shut down the machine when activated.

Air embolism is characterized by the sudden onset of severe hypotension, breathlessness, cyanosis, and collapse. A loud precordial murmur is audible on oscillation. When significant volumes of air have entered the circulation, subsequent pulmonary vascular obstruction and respiratory failure have generally resulted in the patient's death.[16,17] To prevent death from occurring when air embolism is present or suspected, the infusion tubing should be clamped off and the patient immediately turned onto his or her left side in a prone position. This prevents air in the right ventricle from entering the pulmonary arterial outflow.

**Hypothermia**

The administration of relatively large amounts of cold blood, transported directly from the blood bank refrigerator to the recipient without prewarming, is most likely to produce problems when the volume administered is large relative to the total blood volume of the patient. Thus, massive cold blood transfusion may produce various adverse results in the following situations: trauma resuscitation; high-volume replacement in surgery; and the exchange transfusion of newborns. When massive cold blood transfusions (10°C–13°C) have been given to adult patients, considerable cooling of intraesophageal temperatures (as low as 27.5°C) has been recorded.[18,19] Ventricular cardiac arrhythmias are observed rather frequently in surgical patients transfused with relatively large volumes of unwarmed blood.[20-22]

A low temperature increases the left-shift produced in the oxygen-hemoglobin dissociation curve. This results from the depletion of 2, 3-diphosphoglycerate (2, 3-DPG) observed in RBCs that are stored for longer than 7 days in CPD or CPD-A1. When cold blood is administered on other biochemical parameters (eg, plasma levels of glucose and the hormones involved in carbohydrate metabolism, such as insulin, glucagon, growth hormone, etc) it appears to have little effect. There is some impairment of citrate metabolism, and systemic cooling may be expected to impair the synthesis rate of some procoagulants.[23] Routine warming of blood is strongly recommended in the treatment of patients who have cold-type hemolytic anemia, cold agglutinin disease or paroxysmal cold hemoglobinuria, and for the exchange transfusion of newborns.

### Transfusion of Foreign and Particulate Material

The development and consequences of transfusion of microaggregates in stored blood products have already been discussed. The use of disposable plastic tubing, harnesses, and properly constructed filtration devices in modern transfusion equipment has almost eliminated the risk of blood product contamination by other particulate materials. Prior to the development of these devices, occasional problems were encountered when the use of resterilizable rubber tubing, glass bottles, and loosely constructed filters would permit small particles of rubber, glass, or cellulose fibers to enter the circulation.

Fat embolism, most often seen in major skeletal trauma, is a somewhat rare complication of intramedullary transfusion. Occasional embolization of intravenous catheters has been described to require surgical removal.[24,25] Such accidents can be avoided by the use of catheters that are advanced intravenously over guide wires or by needles with properly over-fitting catheters.

Plasticizers, particularly phthalates, have been associated with measurable levels of fat embolism both in blood plasma and in body fat after transfusion. Varying degrees of toxicity have been attributed to their use. In particular, diminished RBC survival and platelet dysfunction have resulted from association with these substances. Recent advances in the manufacture of blood bags that do not require plasticizers have permitted the use of plastics that are of greater resilience and permeability than gases. These improvements have largely eliminated the potential for toxicity problems.[26,27]

## Metabolic, Biochemical, and Hemostatic Problems of Transfusion

### Citrate Toxicity and Hypocalcemia

Rapid administration of large volumes of blood or blood products containing citrate anticoagulant-preservative solutions can produce significant elevations of plasma citrate levels. These can reach to 1000-fold the upper limit of normal.[28] Elevated citrate levels produce adverse effects primarily by chelating ionized calcium. This action produces the symptoms and signs of hypocalcemia that are most likely to occur when large volumes of cold blood are administered rapidly, as in trauma resuscitation, major surgery with compensation of high-volume blood loss, and in the exchange transfusion of newborns. Administration of significant quantities of cold blood may produce sufficient overall body cooling to reduce markedly the metabolism of citrate by the liver. Again, patients with hepatocellular disease or significant biliary obstruction will exhibit citrate toxicity more readily than normal persons after smaller amounts blood product have been transfused.[29-31]

The clinical manifestations of citrate toxicity match those of hypocalcemia: increased neuromuscular sensitivity with involuntary twitching and ultimately tetany with carpopedal spasm; circumoral and other paraesthesia; cardiac arrhythmias and abnormal ECG findings; abnormal QRS complexes; and S-T segment prolongation. Cardiac output may be diminished, and, in severe cases that are not promptly treated, resultant ventricular fibrillation may cause death. These symptoms and signs of hypocalcemia resulting from excessive administration of citrate are rapidly reversed by the intramuscular (or, in severe cases, intravenous) administration of calcium gluconate or calcium chloride.

Prophylaxis with calcium should be given where large amounts of blood are to be replaced at a rapid rate, as in massive transfusion or in exchange transfusions (where 2 blood volumes are to be replaced in 2 hours or less). The usual suggested dose is 4.5 mEq of calcium per liter of blood, used or exchanged. The 4.5 mEq of ionized calcium is provided by 10 mL of 10% calcium gluconate or 2.4 mL of 10% calcium chloride. In patients with significant hepatic dysfunction or in whom delay in citrate metabolism can be anticipated, it is sometimes difficult to assess the amount of calcium necessary to guard against toxicity or its reversal once developed. In such cases, caution should be observed with regard to the dosage of calcium administered. Also, careful, constant monitoring of the patient should be undertaken, including electrocardiographic telemetry and the frequent measurement of plasma-ionized calcium levels.

**Hyperkalemia**

Adenosine triphosphate (ATP) levels within the RBC gradually decline during storage at 1°C to 6°C, most particularly in ACD- or CPD-stored blood or RBCs, since the building blocks for successful regeneration of purine nucleotides are not provided in these solutions. As energy-rich phosphate bonds of ATP become less and less available in such circumstances, the cell membrane pump mechanism, an energy-dependent active transport system mediated through a Na+/K–activated ATPase, becomes progressively less effective. Sodium ions begin to diffuse into the RBC along their concentration gradient, together with their hydration "envelope" of water molecules. Likewise, as the stored RBCs become increasingly spherocytic and hyperhydrated, there is a concurrent outward diffusion of K+ ions into the extracellular plasma, again along their concentration gradient. This loss is about 1 mEq/day/unit, at least during approximately the first week of storage. After 7 days, a plasma potassium concentration of about 11 mEq/L may be observed. At 2 weeks, this value will be approximately 20 mEq/L. At 3 weeks, values of 30 to 35 mEq/L may be seen. The situation is less acute with more modern anticoagulant-preservative solutions, which incorporate adenine as well as inorganic phosphate and glucose. These concentrations are able to maintain better ATP levels in the stored RBCs and enable liquid storage to be continued for as long as 35 to 42 days. A unit stored in CPD-A1 for 35 days is comparable to an ordinary CPD-stored unit at 21 days' shelf life as far as the plasma level of potassium is concerned.

Transfusions of hyperkalemic RBCs, even when large volumes are administered in trauma resuscitation or certain surgical procedures, are unlikely to produce significant adverse effects unless the patient already shows hyperkalemia or has significant impairment of renal function. Occasionally, however, cardiac arrhythmias or even cardiac arrest might be influenced by such large doses of potassium, particularly when concomitant citrate toxicity and hypothermia combine and reinforce the effect. This appears to be a rare occurrence in humans.

It is questionable whether, theoretically, the adverse effects of hyperkalemia are as dangerous a risk to the patient as the incipient hypoxia and metabolic acidosis (with its attendant organ damage) that accompany severe and prolonged hypovolemic shock.[32] Again, the use of RBC concentrates rather than whole blood greatly reduces the volume of plasma transfused and therefore the amount of potassium given. It does seem reasonable to avoid the administration of excessive amounts of components that contain high levels of potassium, especially when the patient is initially hyperkalemic or shows impaired renal function.

## Reactions Associated With Vasoactive Substances

It is uncommon for reactions to occur where they relate specifically to the release of vasoactive substances in stored, nonbacterially contaminated blood components. The possible dysrhythmic effects of citrate and potassium have already been discussed, as well as the potential effects of allergic and anaphylactoid reactions on blood pressure. Most other constituents of anticoagulant-preservative solutions are innocuous in the concentrations used under clinical circumstances. Levels of adenine greater than those found in current proprietary preparations can be toxic and could cause hypotensive responses. Its presence, however, is not observed with licensed adenine-containing preservative solutions.

Occasional hypotensive reactions, severe in some instances, have been observed with both fresh frozen plasma (FFP) and certain plasma derivatives, including plasma protein fraction (PPF) and very rarely 5% human plasma albumin.[33] In these reported cases, prekallikrein activator (PKA) in the parent plasma appeared to have undergone activation during processing and was carried over in a significant amount into the final product. Transfusion of such material into a recipient may bring about the activation of the plasma-kinin pathway, converting prekallikrein to kallikrein. This in turn will cause the generation of bradykinin from an inert circulating decopeptide kininogen. Rapid generation of large quantities of bradykinin may create a significant and sometimes severe hypotensive reaction. However, most of these reactions are transient, since rapid inactivation of bradykinin by kininase is generally observed, particularly in the pulmonary circulation. Modification of the fractionation techniques used for production of PPF and human albumin for transfusion have eliminated this problem. Similar effects have been observed with freshly thawed FFP in patients who are undergoing cardiopulmonary bypass surgery.[34,35] Freezing of freshly drawn plasma in some units appears to facilitate the activation of PKA, with subsequent generation of bradykinin either in the unit itself or within the recipient after transfusion. Rather severe hypotensive reactions can be observed in some patients who are undergoing cardiopulmonary bypass surgery. These may be attributed to the fact that, in cases in which the pulmonary circulation is temporarily bypassed, inactivation of bradykinin is retarded, and the effects of this substance are therefore more persistent. Pressor agents such as dopamine might be necessary to counteract the bradykinin effect on certain patients.

Transfusion of multiple units of RBCs has occasionally been associated with a severe hypertensive reaction (accompanied by a sharp rise in blood pressure, vasoconstriction, convulsions, and sometimes fatal cerebral hemorrhage) in patients with sickle-cell anemia and thalassemia major.[36-38] This development has been difficult to explain in the reported cases. Mechanical factors such as circulatory overload have generally been excluded, and a pressor agent affecting vascular tone and peripheral resistance appears to be more likely. Generation of angiotensin has been suggested but not proven.

## Iron Overload

Inappropriate accumulation of iron in various parts of the body is a well-recognized complication of long-term transfusion therapy with RBC concentrates and is primarily treatable with hemotherapy. These include thalassemia major, sickle-cell anemia and other hemoglobinopathies, myelodysplastic disorders, primary RBC dysplasia, aplastic anemia of varying etiology, congenital atransferrinemia, and some cases of chronic renal failure with associated anemia of chronic disease.

A unit of RBCs contains some 200 mg of iron. Frequent administration of RBC transfusions over a period of years therefore inevitably leads to accumulation of iron within the body. Excretion of this metal is extremely difficult. Women are at some advantage over men in this context because they are able to eliminate some iron during their menstrual cycle. Nevertheless, menstrual discharge is often insufficient to compensate for the continued incremental iron buildup created by chronic transfusion. Some patients may show increased uptake of iron, in addition to the considerable load produced by repeated transfusion, further complicating the situation. Thus, in patients with either thalassemia major or sideroblastic anemia, there is definite evidence of increased iron absorption from the alimentary tract, which adds further to these patients' difficulties.[39-41]

Iron overload produced by transfusion may be a relatively innocuous process. It has been suggested that much of the iron found in macrophages of the reticuloendothelial system is stored relatively harmlessly, whereas iron overload produced by excessive absorption from the alimentary tract, as in hemochromatosis, leads to parenchymal iron deposition with pathologic effects. There is some measure of truth in this observation. Continued iron loading through chronic transfusion can also produce well-defined adverse effects on various organs.

The distinction between hemosiderosis and hemochromatosis is obscured when one considers long-term RBC therapy for severe chronic anemia. Parenchymal deposits of iron in the myocardium, the conducting system of the heart, the liver, the pancreas, and the gonads have been noted. Thus, the following occurrences have been described: cardiac arrhythmias with eventual overt failure; hepatic dysfunction with varying degrees of fibrosis; pancreatic fibrosis with variable occurrence of diabetes mellitus; and growth retardation in children accompanied by delayed sexual development.[42] Serum iron levels and serum keratin levels are elevated, while their iron-binding capacity is generally saturated or nearly saturated. For patients undergoing long-term transfusion therapy, the following are indicated periodically: careful screening of the heart, including tests of mechanical performance and ECG; liver biopsy for evidence of iron deposition and fibrosis; and evaluation of pancreatic endocrine function for evidence of diabetes. The management of established transfusion-related hemosiderosis is unsatisfactory. Clearly in these cases, unlike the situation in hereditary hemochromatosis, removal of iron by repeated phlebotomy is not possible. Use of the compound desferrioxamine, an iron-chelating agent, by daily intramuscular injection has not produced satisfactory results, and other iron-chelating agents, especially those administered by the oral route, have been ineffective to date. Again, substances that have been introduced to complex iron in the alimentary tract to reduce absorption have had little effect on the development of iron-related complications in patients with thalassemia major. While some benefit has been claimed for the oral administration of tannate in reducing iron absorption in thalassemia,[43] on the whole it must be regarded as less than satisfactory. Patients should be advised to avoid iron-containing foods, or the overall results of this conservatism on the development of transfusion hemosiderosis is questionable.

In young children with thalassemia major, some benefit may be obtained from the use of young RBCs (neocytes) obtained from whole blood units by differential centrifugation and concentration. Unquestionably, the mean survival time of such cells is significantly longer than the average survival time in the circulation of an average donor RBC. The regular use of neocyte-rich RBC preparations definitely prolongs the intervals between transfusions.[42-46] The cost, however, is extremely high and because of this, and the number of units necessary to produce sufficient neocyte-rich material for transfusion, this method is rendered unrealistic and thus of little value in older children or adolescents.

## Defects of Hemostasis in Massive Transfusion

The principal source of hemostatic defects in patients receiving large quantities of blood components, particularly stored whole blood or RBCs, is thrombocytopenia. In such patients, this condition may have a complex origin in which several factors are involved.

1) Extensive tissue injury may occur in trauma cases, which may in turn activate consumption of platelets at those sites of injury as part of the physiologic hemostatic response.
2) Large amounts of blood may be lost, thereby reducing or eliminating platelets by hemorrhage.
3) Development of varying degrees of disseminated intravascular coagulation (DIC) is common in patients with multiple injuries, which in turn leads to further platelet consumption as well as to increased consumption of soluble procoagulants.
4) The possible presence of platelet-aggregating factors in stored plasma products and the consumption of platelets by passive involvement with transfused microaggregate debris may contribute to thrombocytopenia to some extent.[46,47]
5) Replacement of the patient's depleted blood volume with large amounts of stored blood, RBCs containing few or no viable platelets, or "washout" thrombocytopenia, is directly proportional to the volume of platelet-depleted blood or product transfused.[48]

The hemorrhagic diathesis associated with thrombocytopenia is particularly characterized by continued oozing of blood from puncture sites, suture lines, and wounds. In all cases where bleeding appears excessive, it is imperative to determine whether or not the patient has a leaking blood vessel that needs to be located and secured, rather than merely assuming that significant degrees of hemorrhage are the result of thrombocytopenia. In general, the thrombocytopenia produced by dilution is unlikely to lead to significant and serious bleeding when the platelet count is in excess of $50 \times 10^9$/L (50,000/$mm^3$). On the other hand, while it is well recognized that patients who have been receiving extracorporeal circulation with use of an oxygenator may have relatively high platelet counts, the qualitative function of the circulating platelets may also be variously impaired. In such cases, platelet transfusions may have to be considered in patients whose postoperative platelet count is 50 x $10^9$/L (50,000/$mm^3$) or even higher. This issue is even further complicated in the presence of DIC when treatment may necessarily require other components (fresh frozen plasma, cryoprecipitate) to expedite treatment for a genuine consumptive coagulopathy.

Insofar as dilutional thrombocytopenia is concerned, the degree of thrombocytopenia is directly proportional to the volume of stored blood transfused, and therefore also proportional to the dilutional effect on the patient's own platelets. Thus, it should be fairly easy to predict at which point platelet transfusions must be administered to patients receiving massive transfusions, provided that the initial pretransfusion platelet count has been determined. This process should always be part of the baseline work-up of such cases.[49] Platelet concentrates are the components of choice for management of dilutional thrombocytopenia and should be given in sufficient amount to maintain a circulating platelet count of greater than 50 x $10^9$/L (50,000/$mm^3$). Generally, 6 pooled single-donor platelet units (or 1 "6-pack" of platelets) obtained by apheresis may be administered for every 10 units of blood replaced. The prophylactic use of fresh whole blood in these circumstances is not often a practical possibility. Unless transfused fairly promptly (within 12 hours of collection), efficacy is questionable. In most instances, such units are not obtainable since they will not have had, in most instances, all the requisite testing for infectious agents completed during that time. The use of platelet concentrates is strongly recommended in this situation.

So-called "wash-out" coagulopathy, due to the dilution of coagulation factors (as distinct from platelets), is probably of much less significance in the context of massive transfusion. Most soluble procoagulants maintain normal or close to normal levels during storage at 1°C to 6°C, but the labile factors V and VIII deteriorate during storage. In particular, factor VIII levels fall by about 50% of their initial activity in the first 24 hours of shelf life. Although factor V declines more slowly, both are significantly depleted after 7 to 10 days of storage, as compared to their initial values. It should be pointed out that normal coagulated functions may be maintained with activities of these labile soluble procoagulants as low as 20% of normal. It is, therefore, questionable whether massive transfusions of bank blood ever deplete the circulating activities of these factors below a level consistent with normal coagulative function. It could be speculated that patients with multiple injuries and extensive tissue injury consume procoagulants at an accelerated rate and that some degree of significant depletion may be achieved in these instances if replacement therapy with stored blood is given exclusively. However, by comparison with potential effects of thrombocytopenia, dilutional effects on coagulation factor levels are of less importance.[50-52] Coagulation factor levels can be the periodic inclusion of a unit of fresh frozen plasma for every 7 to 8 units replaced.

The presence of an active consumptive coagulopathy (DIC) may result in serious depletion of a wide range of procoagulants and thereby require necessary additional therapy with cryoprecipitate (factor VIII and fibrinogen), factor IX complex, and platelets, in addition to fresh frozen plasma, may be necessary to overcome the consumptive process.[53]

## Problems Associated With Exchange Transfusion of Newborns

Traditionally, the management of severe hemolytic disease of the newborn (HDN) is the most important indication for whole blood exchange transfusion of newborns. However, other indications may include neonatal respiratory distress, neonatal sepsis, and hyperbilirubinemia. The problems associated with this process resemble those of massive transfusion but are generally less severe and more readily controlled. The principal risks characteristic with the process are as follows:

1) Appropriate selection of the component used for performing exchange transfusion can go a long way toward averting some of the biochemical difficulties encountered in past years. For example, the discontinuance of acid citrate dextrose as a standard anticoagulant preservative for whole blood and RBCs has largely eliminated the risk of metabolic acidosis, which was periodically observed, particularly in the exchange transfusion of small premature neonates (those weighing less than 1500 g). With modern preservative solutions, this is no longer a hazard. Hyperkalemia can similarly be avoided by using either whole blood less than 5 days old or reconstituted whole blood composed of frozen, deglycerolyzed RBCs reconstituted with fresh frozen plasma, with the hematocrit of the final product adjusted appropriately. Electrolyte levels in these products are normal.

2) Blood for exchange transfusion should be drawn in CPD, CPD-A1, or AS-1 anticoagulant preservative solutions. Heparin should be avoided because the heparin content of an average unit is many times the "heparinizing dose" for an infant. It must therefore be regarded as potentially dangerous if used in this application. Citrate toxicity (ie, symptoms and signs attributable to citrate chelation of ionized calcium) can be avoided by the routine prophylactic use of calcium gluconate.

3) Since life-threatening hypothermia can develop during or after exchange transfusion of newborns, particularly when they are performed rapidly (less than 2 hours' duration), blood used in exchange transfusions should be prewarmed in a 37°C waterbath

before administration. In the case of smaller premature infants, a blood warmer may be incorporated in the circuit.

4) Care should be taken to fill all parts of the tubing to be used in the system with fluid before introducing an intravenous catheter through the umbilical vein (or parenteral vein when necessary) to eliminate the risk of air embolism in the system. This condition results from the introduction of an intravenous catheter, which contains air, through the umbilical vein and into the ductus venosus, where there is a negative pressure that may serve to aspirate air into the circulation.[54] Such occurrences can be avoided by ensuring that the catheter is filled with fluid (eg, normal saline) before it is inserted. A similar occurrence has been documented for catheters in a subdiaphragmatic position.[55]

5) Care should be taken when inserting the catheter to avoid creating a false passage or rupturing the umbilical vein. If resistance to passage of the catheter is encountered, it should be withdrawn. A new attempt should then be made to insert it with care, never advancing the tip forcibly against resistance. Location of the correct passage is indicated by ease of forward movement and by the appearance of blood in the catheter when gentle suction is applied by means of an attached syringe. It is as well to advance the catheter so that the tip passes into the inferior vena cava of the infant, where flow problems are usually not encountered.

6) Since many infants may show an elevated venous pressure, especially those with severe hemolytic disease of the newborn and concomitant cardiac failure, a measurement of this pressure should first be taken using a suitable monometer with an aliquot of blood withdrawn to reduce this pressure initially. The transfusion should then follow slowly. Circulatory overload will be avoided by removing more blood than is replaced. Customarily, the equivalent of 2 blood volumes is exchanged for hemolytic disease of the newborn, neonatal sepsis, and respiratory distress syndrome.

With respect to large molecular species or particulate elements such as RBCs, it can be shown that a residual percentage of the patient's own indigenous components remaining after various volumes of blood have been exchanged is given by the following formula:

$$R(\%) = \frac{[v - s]^n}{v} \times 100$$

R = residual percentage of the element being considered (eg, RBCs, plasma protein molecules, etc); v = infant's blood volume in mL; s = volume in mL of each aliquot exchanged; and n = total number of aliquots exchanged.

When the total volume exchanged is equal to a single infant blood volume, then R is approximately 33%. When 2 blood volumes are exchanged, R becomes about 11%, and when 3 volumes are exchanged, R becomes approximately 3.5%. A single-volume exchange clearly does not achieve as good a result as a 2-volume exchange, which can be accomplished in approximately 2 to 2.5 hours. A 3-volume exchange is a long and tedious procedure and very exhausting for the infant patient, relative to the little additional gain in total exchange. Two-volume exchanges are thus preferred as routine procedures rather than 1-volume or 3-volume operations.

## Special Risks of Therapeutic Plasma Exchange, Photapheresis, and Related Technology

Centrifugal apheresis is a technology that has reached a high level of sophistication. It is used extensively, both to prepare cellular and liquid blood components and to carry out therapeutic plasma exchange. A minor modification of this technique is also used in the process of "photapheresis" in which a fluorophore (psoralen) is administered to a patient with certain proliferative disorders (eg, cutaneous T-cell lymphoma) and in certain autoimmune conditions (eg, scleroderma). Leukocyte-rich plasma is then separated by centrifugal apheresis, and the leukocyte suspension is then subjected to appropriate ultraviolet (UV) light irradiation. The UV irradiation brings about photoactivation of the fluorophore, which then interacts with the DNA of the neoplastic T cells. This process inhibits their replication and eventually causes their destruction. After irradiation, the leukocytes and plasma are returned to the patient.

An increasing number of disorders, particularly autoimmune disorders, are being treated by therapeutic plasma exchange (TPE). The principal hazards associated with these methodologies are as follows:

1) Local complications include hematomas at the venipuncture sites and occasionally superficial venous thrombosis. Infection of such sites is rarely observed and should not occur if proper preparative techniques are used prior to insertion of needles or catheters.

2) Hypovolemic hypotension is occasionally observed when significant volumes of blood are outside of the patient's circulation at any one time. This condition is more likely to develop when intermittent-flow devices are used as opposed to modern, continuous-flow devices. With the use of the latter device, total extracorporeal volume is generally very small, and steady-state kinetics of blood flow is maintained. Hypotensive attacks are likely to be most troublesome in patients with neurologic disorders who are undergoing therapeutic plasma exchange, particularly for conditions in which dysautonomia is likely to be a frequent complication (Guillain-Barré syndrome, multiple sclerosis, and other types of polyneuropathy). Such patients may exhibit

significant vascular instability as a result of their dysautonomia. Exaggerated hypotensive responses may sometimes occur even with relatively small extracorporeal volumes of blood. This situation must be responded to promptly by rapid volume correction.

3) Citrate toxicity and hypocalcemia are most likely to be encountered in preparative thrombocytopheresis and TPE in which significant volumes of citrate-containing fluids are mixed with the patient's circulating blood. Circumoral tingling, other paraesthesias, and neuromuscular hyposensitivity may occur. The prophylactic use of calcium in these cases will obviate this complication.

4) Allergic-anaphylactoid reactions to plasma, including urticaria, erythematous reactions, wheezing and bronchospasm, and, occasionally, anaphylaxis, may complicate the administration of plasma products during these procedures. The etiology and circumstances of such reactions are the same as those discussed in the context of regular transfusion. Management consists of terminating the procedure and appropriately administering antihistamines for allergic reactions. Both severe reactions and anaphylactic responses will require intensive management with epinephrine and pressor agents.

5) Leukocytopheresis, used for the preparation of granulocytes, involves the use of hydroxyethyl starch (HES) as a sedimenting agent to effect clean separation between RBCs and granulocytes. Because HES is an efficient plasma expander, capable of increasing plasma volume quickly, the process may be sufficiently rapid to manifest itself with headache and occasionally the development of peripheral edema. However, the condition is self-limiting since the HES is excreted through the kidneys at a predictable rate, and the problem is corrected by the accompanying diuresis. Allergic reactions to HES, generally urticarial in nature, are occasionally seen. They can be complicated by bronchospasm. If this condition occurs, the procedure should be terminated and antihistamines administered.[56]

6) Hypersensitivity reactions to heparin or protamine have been described. Chills, urticarial rashes, bronchospasm, and even genuine anaphylaxis may occur but are fortunately rare. A bleeding diathesis may result from inappropriate administration of heparin.[57] The occurrence of any of these reactions mandates both the immediate discontinuance of the procedure and treatment of the specific reaction with appropriate therapy (eg, antihistamines, epinephrine, etc) as the case demands.

7) Air embolism as a potential complication of apheresis procedures or therapeutic plasma exchange is very rare. It is essential, however, before beginning such a procedure to ascertain that all tubing and connections to be used in the procedure are properly filled with fluid

and free of air. Most apheresis devices currently in use are amply provided with air-bubble traps on the return lines to the patient as well as electronic sensors that respond to air bubbles or to obstructions to flow within the system. If either occurs, the device will automatically sound a warning and shut down the machine. As a result, this complication has been virtually eliminated.

Photapheresis was introduced relatively recently by Edelson et al[58] as a definitive modality of treatment for systemically disseminated cutaneous T-cell lymphoma (CTCL). This disease is relatively resistant to both chemotherapy and radiotherapy but appears to respond positively to photoactivated 8-methoxy psoralen (8-MOP). The photoactivated product is able to interact with the DNA of the tumor cells separated extracorporeally by apheresis, which results in blockage of replication and ultimately to the death of the cells. The drug is given orally in a dose sufficient to produce a blood level of 50 mg/dL, which is achieved about 2 hours after the oral dose. At this time, a lymphocyte-rich faction of blood is separated by centrifugal apheresis, then exposed in a special chamber to ultraviolet A (UVA) light (1–2 J/cm$^2$). The product is then reinfused into the patient/donor. This combination of 8-MOP activated by UVA brings about an 88% ± 5% devitalization of the exposed lymphocytes. While exposure to 8-MOP alone is ineffective, this technique appears to provide a valuable clinical adjunct to the management of this disease, and it is relatively free of significant side effects.

Some side effects, however, have been noted, such as intratransfusion or posttransfusion febrile reactions. These generally follow the reinfusion of the irradiated cells and comprise a spike of fever (1°C–3°C), with chills lasting for 8 to 12 hours. In most reported cases, resolution has been completed within 24 hours of onset. Urticarial or angioedematous skin reactions occasionally accompany these febrile episodes. In the series of Edelson et al,[58] such responses were noted only in patients who showed a significant clinical response to treatment. Further treatments following a noticeable response were not accompanied by these reactions. Transient elevation in liver enzymes, without hyperbilirubinemia, has also been occasionally reported. These findings disappear after a short interval.

The few other adverse effects reported during the use of this technology typify those already described for any form of apheresis therapy. They include minor local complications such as hematomas at venipuncture sites, superficial vein thrombosis, and occasionally mild hypovolemic hypotensive reactions. The methodology used in this technology does not appear to pose any particular additional risks to those receiving treatment. At the same time, the patient has the potential for significant advancement in the management phase of an otherwise aggressive and intractable disease. Psoralen will greatly increase cutaneous sensitivity to sunlight by virtue of the readiness with which it will absorb and become activated by ultraviolet light. Therefore, those patients who receive it should be protected against sunlight or serious cutaneous photosensitivity, because burning may occur.

It is likely that photapheresis will find wider application in the future. Currently, the licensed therapeutic application of this technology is confined to the management of selected cases of CTCL, but clinical trials are in progress now to determine its usefulness in systemic sclerosis, intractable psoriasis, dermatomyositis, and in some cases of AIDS. Results of these trials may prove interesting. They may lead to a much wider application of this technique, which has already produced dramatic effects in an otherwise refractory and devastating disease.

## REFERENCES

1. Duke M, Herbert VV, Abelman WH. Hemodynamic effects of blood transfusion in chronic anemia. N Engl J Med. 1964;271:975.
2. Swank RL. Alteration of blood on storage: measurement of adhesiveness of aging platelets and leukocytes and their removal by filtration. N Engl J Med. 1961;265:728.
3. Marshall B, Elison N, Wurzel HA, et al. Microaggregate formation in stored blood, III: influence of anticoagulants in blood components. Circ Shock. 1975;2:185.
4. Arrington A, MacNamara JJ. Mechanism of microaggregate formation in stored blood. Ann Surg. 1974;179:146.
5. Wright G, Sanderson JM. ACD and CPD blood preservation. Lancet. 1974;2:173.
6. Solis RT, Goldfinger D, Gibson ME, et al. Characteristics of microaggregates in stored blood. Transfusion. 1974;40:538.
7. MacNamara JJ, Molot M, Stremple JF. Screen filtration pressure in combat casualties. Ann Surg. 1970;172:334.
8. MacNamara JJ. Microaggregates in stored blood: physiologic significance. In: Chaplin H, Jaffe ER, Lenfant C, et al, eds. Preservation of Red Blood Cells. Washington, DC: National Academy of Sciences; 1973:315.
9. Reul GJ, Bell AC, Greenberg D. Protection of the pulmonary microvasculature by fine screen blood filtration. Chest. 1974;66:4.
10. Dhubramdhar HM, Brown AC, Barrett J, et al. Pulmonary structural changes following microembolism and blood transfusion. Arch Pathol Lab Med. 1979;103:335.
11. Rosario MD, Rumsey EW, Arakaki G, et al. Blood microaggregates and ultrafilters. J Trauma. 1978;18:408.
12. Collins JA, James PM, Bredenderg CE, et al. The relationship between transfusion and hypoxemia in combat casualties. Ann Surg. 1978;188:513.
13. Collins JA. Pulmonary dysfunction and massive transfusion. Bibl Haematol. 1978;46:220.
14. Bredenberg CE. Does a relationship exist between massive blood transfusions and the adult respiratory distress syndrome? If so, what are the best preventative measures? Vox Sang. 1977;32:311.

15. Simpson K. Air accident during transfusion. Lancet. 1942;1:697.

16. Larson CP. Venous air embolism: report of four cases, suggested method of treatment. Am J Clin Pathol. 1951;21:247.

17. Durant TM, Oppenheimer MJ, Lynch PR, et al. Body position in relation to venous air embolism: a roentgenologic study. Am J Med Sci. 1961;265:728.

18. Maclean LD, van Tyn RA. Ventricular defibrillation. JAMA. 1961;175:471.

19. Boyan CP, Howard WS. Cardiac arrest and the temperature of bank blood. JAMA. 1963;183:58.

20. Boyan CP. Cold or warmed blood after massive transfusions. Ann Surg. 1964;160:282.

21. Dubkjaer E, Elkier P. The use of heated blood in massive blood replacement. Acta Anaesthesiol Scand. 1964;8:271.

22. Shapiro M. Safer exchange transfusions with citrated blood. Stockholm: Communication of the 10th Congress of the International Society of Blood Transfusion; 1964.

23. Milner RDG, Feket M, Hodge JS, et al. Influence of donor blood temperature on hyperbolic and hormonal changes during exchange transfusion. Arch Dis Chld. 1972;47:933.

24. Bennett PJ. The use of intravenous plastic catheters. Br Med J. 1963;2:1252.

25. Taylor FW, Rutherford CE. Accidental loss of plastic tube into venous system. Arch Surg. 1963;6:177.

26. Gulbring D. The use of plastics in blood transfusion equipment with special regard to toxicity problems. Vox Sang. 1964;9:513.

27. Marcel YL, Noel SP. Contamination of blood stored in plastic packs. Lancet. 1970;1:35.

28. Weksler IB, Pinkus JD, Natelson S, et al. The fate of citrate in erythoblastotic infants treated with exchange transfusion. J Clin Invest. 1949;28:474.

29. Ludbrok J, Vyan V. Citrate intoxication: a clinical and experimental study. Br Med J. 1958;2:523.

30. Taylor WC, Gillis CN, Nash CW, et al. Experimental observations on cardiac arrhythmia during exchange transfusion in rabbits. J Pediatr. 1961;58:470.

31. Bunker JP, Stetson JB, Coe RC, et al. Citric acid intoxication. JAMA. 1955;157:1361.

32. Melrose DG, Wilson AO. Intra-arterial transfusion: the potassium hazard. Lancet. 1953;1:126.

33. Anstall HB. Adverse reactions to transfusion. In: Anstall HB, Urie PM, eds. A Manual of Hemotherapy. New York, NY: John Wiley and Sons; 1986:341-360.

34. Huggins C. Personal communication; 1984.

35. Cederhaum AI, Roberts HR. Complications of the use of prothrombin complex concentrates in liver disease. Clin Res. 1973;21:92.

36. Breen F, Tillus JL. Prothrombin concentrates in treatment of Christmas disease and allied disorders. JAMA. 1969;208:1848.

37. Gershwin ME, Gude JK. Deep vein thrombosis and pulmonary embolism in congenital factor VIII deficiency. N Engl J Med. 1973;288:141.

38. Kasper CK. Postoperative thrombosis in Hemophilia B. N Engl J Med. 1973;289:160.

39. Bothwell T, Finch CA. Iron Metabolism. London: Churchill-Livingstone; 1962:410.

40. Weatherall DJ. Protein synthesis in the red cell: the thalassaemias and related disorders. In: Hardisty RM, Weatherall DJ, eds. Blood and its Disorders. Oxford: Blackwell Scientific; 1974:630.

41. Modell CB. Transfusional hemochromatosis. In: Kief H, ed. Iron Metabolism and its Disorders. Amsterdam: Excerpta Medica; 1975:230.

42. Barton JC. Noninfectious transfusion reactions. In: Dutcher JP, ed. Modern Transfusion Therapy. Boca Raton, Fla: CRC Press; 1990:73-74.

43. de Alarcon PA, Conovan ME, Forbes GB, et al. Iron absorption in the thalassemia syndrome and its inhibition by pea. N Engl J Med. 1979;300:5.
44. Piomell S, Seaman C, Reibman J, et al. Separation of young red cells with improved survival in vivo: an approach to chronic transfusion therapy. Proc Natl Acad Sci USA. 1978;75:3474.
45. National Institutes of Health. Use of neocytes decreases frequency of transfusions to reduce iron overload. JAMA. 1979;142:2669.
46. Propper RD, Button LN, Nathan DG. New approaches to the transfusion management of thalassemia. Blood. 1980;55:55.
47. Jennevine EP, Krevans JR. Mechanism of thrombocytopenia that follows multiple whole blood transfusions. Trans Assoc An Physiol. 1956;69:155.
48. Krevans JR, Jackson DP. Hemorrhagic disorder following massive whole blood transfusions. JAMA. 1955;159:171.
49. Noe DA, Graham SM, Luff R, et al. Platelet counts during rapid massive transfusion. Transfusion. 1982;22:392.
50. Zucker MB, Sigel M, Clifton EE, et al. Generalized excessive oozing in patients undergoing major surgery and receiving multiple blood transfusions. J Lab Clin Med. 1957;50:849.
51. Ingram GIC. The bleeding complications of blood transfusion. Transfusion. 1965;5:1.
52. Miller RD, Robbins TO, Tong MJ, et al. Coagulation defects associated with massive blood transfusion. Ann Surg. 1971;174:794.
53. Barton JC. Massive transfusion: complications and their management. J Tenn Med Assoc. 1975;68:895.
54. van Loghem JJ, van Bolhuis JH, Soeters JM, et al. Treatment of 160 cases of erythroblastosis with heparinized ACD blood. Acta Dis Child. 1974;49:940.
55. Bessis M, Dausset J. Etude critique des remissions au cours des leucemies aigues traties par exsanguines transfusions. Rev Hematol. 1950;5:188.
56. Strauss RG, Kopke JA. Chemistry, pharmacology and donor effects of hydroxyethyl starch as used during leukapheresis. Plasma Ther. 1980;1:35.
57. Urie PM. Apheresis: general considerations. In: Anstall HB, Urie PM, eds. A Manual of Hemotherapy. New York, NY: John Wiley and Sons; 1986:156-170.
58. Edelson R, Berger C, Gaspro F, et al. Treatment of cutaneous T-cell lymphoma by extracorporeal photochemotherapy: preliminary results. N Engl J Med. 1987;316:297.

CHAPTER 7

# GRAFT-VS-HOST DISEASE IN RELATION TO BLOOD TRANSFUSION

## ETIOLOGY AND PATHOGENESIS

It is not our intention here to give an exhaustive review of the different aspects of this subject, but to discuss it primarily as graft-vs-host disease (GVHD), a relatively uncommon but formidable complication of the transfusion of blood and certain blood components. Because of the acknowledged severity of this disorder, it is necessary to discuss in some detail the type of patient most susceptible, the blood components most likely under defined circumstances to lead to the development of this condition after transfusion, and the principles to be employed in its prevention.

Transfusion-related GVHD occurs occasionally in certain recipients whose immune system has become compromised for one reason or another and who have been transfused with blood or blood components containing a "critical mass" of viable lymphocytes. Engraftment of these cells and rejection of them by host tissue results in a most serious and highly lethal disease, which widely involves the skin, gastrointestinal tract, liver, and bone marrow. Graft-vs-host disease occurring in immunosuppressed patients after transfusion is even more aggressive than that following bone marrow transplantation; it is an intense immunologic reaction that is fatal in more than 90% of cases. This reaction is brought about by immunocompetent lymphocytes that are derived from donor blood and become directed against the tissues of the recipient.

An important initial factor in posttransfusion GVHD is the combination of similarity between the HLA antigens of the recipient and those of the donor lymphocytes, and at the same time the presence of some disparity between them. Thus, especially in an immunocompromised host, some degree of similarity between the histocompatibility antigens of the recipient and the donor may be sufficient to permit engraftment of the donor cells within the host. Successful engraftment and proliferation of the environment may permit the rejection of the host by the engrafted cells on the basis of the immunologic differences between the HLA complex of the graft and that of the host.[2] Thus, 2 factors are involved: a degree of similarity in histocompatibility antigenic make-up shared by the host and donor lymphocytes and a degree of disparity in the histocompatibility antigenic make-up between them. This combination in an immunosuppressed patient may enable the grafting multiplication of donor lymphocytes to occur (a function of the similarities between host and graft), while the differences that exist may enable the immunocompetent graft to survive but also to reject the immunocompromised host. In a case reported by Simes and Koskimides,[3] HLA antigenic similarity between the host and the recipient was extremely close, the only noticeable difference being between HLA-B44 in the host and HLA-B38 in the donor. It was concluded that the close similarity between the major histocompatibility make-up of both donor and recipient permitted the successful engraftment of donor lymphocytes. Given the general milieu of immunocompromise in the recipient, this successful action permitted the engrafted donor cells to reject the host tissues in response to recognition of the single antigenic difference between them, as expressed on the recipient's cells.[3]

The several cases reported in the Japanese literature in 1955, together with those described in subsequent studies,[4,5,7,8] were characterized by the rapid onset of an acute illness with fever, diarrhea, erythrodermia, hepatic dysfunction, and, subsequently, bone marrow failure. The disease developed within a variable period after major surgery in which multiple transfusions were given, ranging from a few days to several weeks. This syndrome, first known in Japan and labeled there as postoperative erythrodermia (POE), has been recognized since 1955.[6] Prior to the evolution of the HLA system and our present understanding of it, POE was often ascribed to the adverse effects of certain drugs.[4] In retrospect, however, it appears virtually certain that the syndrome is in reality a form of GVHD, although it apparently occurs in an unimmunocompromised patient population. Most of the earlier cases described were diagnosed in patients undergoing major cardiothoracic surgery, gastrointestinal surgery, or major vascular surgery involving the abdominal aorta. Further inquiry revealed that a majority of patients were elderly and that a number were also receiving significant doses of corticosteroids in the perioperative period. Then, the tendency to use "fresh or nearly fresh" blood in the transfusion of these patients was conspicuous. In this context, the term "fresh" might have been taken to mean blood products that were less than 5 days old and in which it could be shown that lymphocytes remained viable. Clinical evidence suggests that in vitro responsiveness of lymphocytes stored in the temperature range of 1°C to 6°C remains intact for at least 5 days, so that the transfusion of such cells into a recipient who could provide an environment suitable for engraftment (based on antigenic similarity between host and donor) might result in disease. In some cases studied, the similarity between the HLA antigenic make-up of the recipient and the donor has been extremely close, if not identical. In such cases, particularly where some degree of immunosuppression is present (as from moderate dosage of corticosteroids), this similarity may not only permit engraftment of donor cells but may also encourage the subsequent rejection of the host on the basis of disparity between host and donor antigens other than those of the HLA system.

The incidence of these postoperative cases of GVHD has been sufficient to excite a good deal of attention. A survey of 63,257 patients who had undergone cardiac surgery and who had been multiply transfused revealed 96 cases of POE, an incidence of 1 in 660 patients.[9] Undoubtedly, another factor of major significance in the etiology of this condition is the high frequency of occurrence of certain HLA haplotypes among the Japanese population. The incidence of HLA-identical or nearly identical make-up between the recipient of a blood transfusion and the donor providing the component is relatively frequent there. Observations have already been made indicating that a disparity between the engrafted donor cells and the tissues of the recipient may often be based on the presence of antigens that do not belong to the HLA system. In this country and elsewhere, by contrast, host-transfusion GVHD is generally seen in various populations of immunocompromised patients, and the rejection of the host tissues by the graft is most frequently based on the disparity between the HLA antigens of the host and those of the graft.

## Practical Aspects of Posttransfusion Graft-vs-Host Disease

### Patient Groups at Risk

Patients may be divided into the following categories of susceptibility for the development of transfusion-related GVHD: high, intermediate, and low.

#### *High Risk*

In this category are patients who have recently undergone bone marrow transplantation, whether autologous or allogenic,[10,11] and those patients born with either combined-type or cellular-inherited immunologic deficiency.[12-15] In the case of bone marrow transplant recipients, immunosuppression is a deliberate part of the regimen designed to permit the successful acceptance of either bone marrow from an HLA-identical donor or purged autologous marrow (after intensive treatment for hematologic malignancy). An environment is thus created that may not permit the engraftment of HLA-identical bone marrow cells from a donor or the re-engraftment of autologous marrow but may permit the engraftment of viable lymphocyte derived from transfused blood or blood components. As multiple component transfusion therapy is an essential adjunctive treatment modality in these patients, it is clear that they should receive only irradiated products.[16,17]

The other conspicuously high-risk group comprises patients who have inherited immunodeficiency syndromes, particularly the severe combined immunodeficiency syndrome.[13,14,18] This same condition has also been reported after transfusion in patients who have both congenital cellular immunodeficiency and the Wiskott-Aldrich syndrome. Generally, the risk of transfusion-related GVHD appears to be very high among these patients. Even very small numbers of lymphocytes showing minor degrees of HLA disparity with the patient appear to be capable of establishing successful engraftment and host rejection. The literature contains references to patients who have been engrafted by the small number of lymphocytes present in fresh plasma (not fresh frozen plasma), particularly where a 1-haplotype HLA match was present between donor and recipient.[18-20]

### *Intermediate Risk*

Patients at intermediate risk for transfusion-related GVHD include premature newborns who are undergoing whole blood exchange transfusion for hemolytic disease of the newborn (HDN) or for respiratory distress syndrome, particularly where postnatal exchange transfusion has been preceded by intrauterine transfusions. Such cases are usually associated with the use of fresh or relatively fresh whole blood (less than 5 days' shelf life) in which viable lymphocytes can be expected to remain in sufficient numbers to pose a risk for engraftment. The risk seems higher in babies who have received 1 or more intrauterine transfusions with RBC components that contain significant numbers of viable lymphocytes. It has been postulated that this initial exposure to homologous HLA antigens may exhaust the meager resources of the premature immune system, thereby causing an immediate postnatal encounter with viable homologous lymphocytes. The spinoff result may then be toleration of those lymphocytes and subsequent engraftment, followed by rejection of the host.[21-25] The risk appears to diminish with maturity, but the occasional occurrence of this disorder in term babies undergoing exchange transfusion has been reported. The methods of using reconstituted whole blood (frozen deglycerolized RBCs adjusted with fresh frozen plasma) or radiating the product prior to use are both effective in preventing this tragic complication.

Patients with hematologic malignancies are temporarily at intermediate risk for transfusion-related GVHD during the period of marrow suppression and immunologic deficiency, resulting from the chemotherapy necessary to treat the underlying disease. At this time, the use of cellular blood components, particularly platelets, is necessary to sustain the patient through the nadir of chemotherapy. Once there is sufficient recovery of marrow function, the patient can then maintain adequate levels of platelets and an acceptable hematocrit. It is somewhat difficult to assess the magnitude of the risk in these patients; estimates range up to 2% in patients with lymphoma and from 0.1% to 1% in patients with leukemia, in cases involving either adults or children.[26,27] It has been my personal experience that the occurrence of this condition in such patients is infrequent, and I have noted that the risk disappears with recovery of bone marrow and immune function. One might expect that the use of irradiated products for treatment of patients at the nadir of chemotherapy would prevent the condition from occurring; based on this premise, it would follow that these products should thus be considered for treatment of patients receiving HLA-matched platelets obtained by thrombocytopheresis. Currently, however, there is no general recommendation for the exclusive use of irradiated products in patients with leukemia/lymphoma.

The occurrence of transfusion-related GVHD in patients undergoing chemotherapy for solid tumors appears to be rare and has been described in a few patients with neuroblastoma, rhabdomyosarcoma, and glioblastoma. There seems to be a low incidence of this complication appearing in other solid tumors despite therapy and multiple transfusions.[28-32]

### *Low Risk*

In the low-risk category are patients with various disorders in whom a risk of transfusion-related GVHD appears to be a theoretic possibility but is extremely rare in reality. It might be expected that patients with AIDS are especially at risk, but this does not appear to be the case. Despite multiple blood component therapy using nonirradiated components, cases of GVHD associated with AIDS-related transfusions have not, as yet, been reported. Attempts at bone marrow transplantation in AIDS patients have been generally unsuccessful, either having not taken or having shown rapid rejection.[33] Considering the degree of viral-induced immunosuppression that occurs in these patients and their great susceptibility to opportunistic infections with a wide range of organisms (bacterial, protozoal, and fungal) it is indeed surprising that lymphocyte engraftment does not seem to be a problem. Similarly, patients with aplastic anemia who experience bone marrow failure do not appear to be at risk, despite their frequent therapeutic transfusions of cellular blood products. One patient with aplastic anemia who received granulocyte transfusions from a donor with chronic myelocytic leukemia (CML) has been described.[34]

Other patient groups do not appear to be at risk for developing this disorder with the exception of the Japanese patients who developed a form of transfusion-related GVHD (POE) in relation to multiple transfusions during cardiac, gastrointestinal, or vascular surgery, often accompanied by therapeutic modalities that induced varying degrees of immunosuppression.

## Relative Significance of Different Blood Components

By far the most frequent blood component implicated in the development of transfusion-related GVHD is packed red blood cells. Whole blood carries the same theoretic risk but is implicated less often because of the infrequency of its use at the present time.[16] Granulocyte concentrates are probably the next most frequently involved component, with a number of cases reported in which granulocytes were the sole component transfused.[1] Platelets, despite their significant content of viable lymphocytes, have been implicated only rarely as the sole component apparently resulting in the development of transfusion-related GVHD.[26,35] Freshly separated plasma has been the occasional cause of transfusion-related GVHD.[18,19] Fresh frozen plasma (FFP), cryoprecipitate, and frozen deglycerolized RBCs, in which intact lymphocytes may be found in variable numbers have not been reported in association with this condition and thus do not appear to pose a risk, even to immunosuppressed patients, for transfusion-related GVHD.

The occurrence of transfusion-related GVHD in susceptible patients is in many cases dose-related and therefore directly proportional to the number of viable lymphocytes present in a given blood component. Exceptions to this rule may be those high-risk patients with severe, combined congenital immunodeficiency syndrome. In such cases, few homologous lymphocytes may result in successful engraftment and subsequent rejection of the host. In other cases, a reasonably predictable critical mass of lymphocytes appears to be necessary before engraftment is successful and the disease established. Table 7-1 shows the relative lymphocyte content associated with various blood components. In this context, it has been ascertained that a dose of viable lymphocytes equal to or exceeding $10^7$ kg of body weight is required to ensure engraftment. The table will also illustrate that whole blood or packed RBCs contain 1 to 2 x $10^9$ lymphocytes per unit.[36] Based on this, 1 such unit would provide an abundance of lymphocytes to graft a susceptible adult successfully.

In summary, components carrying a high risk include whole blood, packed red blood cells, and granulocyte concentrates. Platelets pose an intermediate risk. To date, frozen deglycerolized RBCs, even when they do appear to have adequate numbers of morphologically identifiable lymphocytes, have not been implicated in transfusion-related GVHD. There is some question as to the viability of these lymphocytes and the degree to which they can be successfully glycerolized to preserve them functionally. Although some lymphocytes may survive, that portion of the total that were originally present may be relatively diminished, resulting in a product that falls below the critical mass of viable lymphocytes likely to produce engraftment. This hypothesis requires confirmation; in the interim, frozen deglycerolized RBCs appear to be a safe product. Fresh plasma that contains only small numbers of lymphocytes is generally considered to be a very low-risk product. It has only caused documented GVHD in occasional cases of severe, combined congenital immunodeficiency syndrome. Frozen plasma and cryoprecipitate contain no morphologically intact lymphocytes and therefore are totally without risk for GVHD.

**TABLE 7-1 LYMPHOCYTE CONTENT OF VARIOUS BLOOD COMPONENTS AND THEIR RELATIVE RISK FOR GRAFT-VS-HOST DISEASE IN A RECIPIENT**

| Component | Number of Lymphocytes per Unit | Risk for GVHD |
|---|---|---|
| Whole blood | 1–2 x $10^9$ | High |
| Packed RBCs (unwashed) | 1–2 x $10^9$ | High |
| Washed RBCs | 6 x $10^7$–$10^8$ | Low |
| Frozen deglycerolized RBCs | Up to 5 x $10^7$ | Very low or none |
| WBC (granulocytes) | 5 x $10^9$ | High |
| Platelets (single-donor unit) | 4 x $10^7$ | Low |
| Platelets (cytapheresis 8-pack) | 3.2 x $10^8$ | Very low |
| Plasma (fresh) | 0 | None |
| Cryoprecipitate | 0 | None |

## Principal Clinical Features

The association of GVHD with bone marrow transplantation has been known for many years and has been observed in experimental animals as well as in humans.[37-40] Graft-vs-host disease following bone marrow transplantation takes 1 of 2 clinical forms: acute or chronic. Typically, the acute form manifests itself between 5 and 10 weeks following the transplantation procedure, whereas the chronic form does not usually appear for at least 15 weeks after transplantation and pursues an indolent course, lasting many months or even years.[41] The acute form of the disease following bone marrow transplantation generally appears some 5 to 10 weeks after the procedure, the initial signs usually being high fever, a widespread erythrodermia, and a complex of symptoms and signs referred to as gastrointestinal dysfunction (nausea and vomiting, severe anorexia, and intractable diarrhea).[42] The cutaneous manifestations are often severe. A diffuse and intense erythema may be complicated by foci, petechiae, or hemorrhagic lesions; other cases show intense local edema with bullous lesions or eventual generalized exfoliation. Envelopment of the liver is indicated by the development of jaundice and variably abnormal liver function tests. This acute form of the disease appears to be mediated primarily by T lymphocytes that are precommitted and have an immunologic memory, rather than stem cells. The disease shows a substantial mortality rate.

The chronic form of this disease does not usually appear until at least 15 weeks after transplantation, and it pursues an indolent course, lasting many months or even years.[41] This variation begins much less conspicuously and is characterized by atrophic and indolent ulcerated skin lesions, exocrine secretory disturbances, gastrointestinal malabsorption, and recurrent pneumonitis.[16,43] The resulting syndrome exhibits many similarities with certain types of autoimmune disease. Special studies for detecting immunoglobulins in affected tissues in chronic GVHD would strongly suggest that the basic mechanism involved is humoral, depending more on immunoglobulin-related mechanisms rather than on T cell–related ones.[42,43]

By contrast, the GVHD that follows blood transfusions in immunosuppressed, susceptible persons shows some striking differences in time of onset, rate of clinical progression, and overall mortality, none of which represent much difference in the pattern of organ involvement. The onset is generally from 5 to 30 days after the transfusion providing the graftable donor cells. The disease progresses to a rapidly fatal conclusion in over 90% of cases. As in bone marrow–related GVHD, the principal organs affected are skin, liver, gastrointestinal tract, and bone marrow. Generally, the form of bone marrow that follows transfusion is much greater and more severe in degree, as distinct from that related to bone marrow transplantation. In the posttransfusion syndrome, engrafted donor cells impinge vigorously on native, autologous bone marrow. This action results in a severe and rapid progression through hypoplasia to aplasia in a majority of cases.[3,44]

This severe and progressive marrow suppression successively leads to pancytopenia, with progressive anemia, leukopenia with its attendant risk of opportunistic infection, and thrombocytopenia. The latter condition may become profound and lead to hemostatic and hemorrhagic complications. It is most often this acute and severe bone marrow failure, generally irreversible, that accounts for the high mortality associated with this condition.

The forms of GVHD following either bone marrow transplantation or transfusion differ also in incidence. In marrow transplantation patients, some manifestations attributable to GVHD occur in as many as 50% to 70% of cases, whereas the occurrence of recognizable GVHD in patients following blood transfusion is very infrequent. Both the clinical course and response to therapy in the 2 situations are also quite different. The disorder after bone marrow transplantation is highly variable; its expression of clinical severity and can be graded from I to IV. Such variations in severity are not generally seen in posttransfusion GVHD, in which virtually all clinical cases fall into the most severe (IV) category. This may, in part, be because the disease in posttransfusion patients is frequently unexpected and may have become well established before it is recognized clinically. However, response to therapy in the posttransfusion form of the disease is abysmal, showing a mortality in excess of 90%. This result contrasts sharply with the events following bone marrow transplantation, in which the mortality is 10% to 20%.

Biopsies of the skin and gastrointestinal mucosa are useful aids in establishing the diagnosis of GVHD. Skin shows edema and intense lymphocytic infiltration, areas of atrophy, basal cell degeneration, and desquamation. Degenerative vascular changes are often present. Similar histologic changes are frequently noted in the gastrointestinal mucosa. Bone marrow biopsy shows marked marrow hypoplasia with intense lymphocytic infiltration. Erythrophagocytosis may be evident. More definitively, transfusion-related GVHD may be discerned in a given patient by demonstrating that most, if not all, circulating lymphocytes are derived from donor sources, rather than from the patient. This has been shown by karyotype analysis and by HLA typing of circulating lymphocytes in the recipient, followed by the process of matching these lymphocytes with those of the donor.[2,3,7,35,45] In such cases, the circulating lymphocytes may have the HLA antigenic make-up of a donor, whereas the antigenic cell structure of the patient's other tissues is characteristic, and thus different.

## Prevention of Transfusion-Related Graft-vs-Host Disease

Prevention of transfusion-related GVHD depends on the recognition and careful clinical examination of patients, focusing on their susceptibility and vulnerability to the possible of lymphocyte engraftment and the avoidance of transfusion involving clinically critical numbers of viable lymphocytes in blood products. Generally speaking, patients with normal immune function are not at risk for posttransfusion GVHD. However, a review of previous material covered indicates that those with varying degrees of immunocompromise are at some risk, and a few patients with special immune deficiencies are at very high risk. Therefore, it is of critical importance to determine initially the risk category to which a given patient belongs before engaging any form of blood transfusion therapy. Some blood products pose a considerable threat to patients who are susceptible, by virtue of immunodeficiency, to GVHD. In particular, whole blood, packed RBCs, and granulocyte concentrates are rich in viable lymphocytes. Between them, they cumulatively account for the overwhelming majority of cases associated with this disorder. Platelet concentrates, which may also contain a significant excess of viable lymphocytes, pose a moderate risk but less than that of whole blood, packed RBCs, and granulocyte concentrates. Simple washing of RBCs does not seem to reduce the number of viable lymphocytes below what might be regarded as a critical mass for immunosuppressed patients. Most often, frozen components, including frozen, deglycerolized RBCs, appear to have little or no potential for causing engraftment.

Careful selection of a component is a primary requirement for the transfusion of patients who fall into high- or moderate-risk categories. The use of irradiated blood products for the transfusion of high-risk patients appears to be the best available safeguard against the subsequent development of transfusion-related GVHD. In this context, it is clear that the dosage of radiation given to the products used is critical; it must be adequate to devitalize sufficient lymphocytes within the products to render them innocuous for the purpose of engraftment.[46]

In assessing the effect of gamma radiation on otherwise viable lymphocytes, 2 parameters in particular have been studied: the response of mixed lymphocyte culture and responses of other lymphocytes to mitogens. In the first instance, a mixed lymphocyte culture response seems to be abolished by relatively small doses of radiation (5 Gy). It might be concluded from this that such a dosage would be adequate to prevent transfusion-related GVHD.[10,47,48] When the response of viable lymphocytes to mitogens is studied, however, a different picture emerges. Thus, in order for radiation to have any productive effect, higher dosages are required: while 15 Gy will reduce the response to mitogens by approximately 85%, a dosage of up to 50 Gy is required to ensure the 98% to 100% suppression of mitogenic response.[49]

A number of studies on various blood components have been undertaken in which these products have been subjected to differing levels of radiation from 5 and 50 Gy, and the results show some variability. In particular, studies of platelet concentrates have indicated that doses of 50 Gy have produced variable results, some claiming no decrease in posttransfusion survival.[49] Other studies have shown increases as high as 33%.[48] The effects on ADP-induced aggregation and collagen-induced aggregation have been variable with doses of 50 Gy.[48-50] Still other studies have indicated that a dose of 50 Gy may cause sufficient platelet damage to reduce or abolish the ability of the irradiated platelets to correct an aspirin-induced prolongation of bleeding time. Reduction of radiation dosage to 20 Gy removed this problem.

Depending on the parameters studied, RBCs seem to be remarkably radioresistant. Very high doses of radiation (100–200 Gy) have virtually no measurable effect on posttransfusion survival of OCr-labeled irradiated RBCs. Such units do not exhibit significant increases in plasma hemoglobin or loss of adenosine triphosphate, 23-diphosphoglycerate. However, some impairment of ion transport function appears to result from radiation levels significantly lower than these. Dosages of 30 Gy are followed by significant leakage of potassium into the surrounding plasma after 24 hours of further storage under normal blood bank conditions. This strongly suggests a degree of RBC functional impairment that is hard to ignore.

Granulocytes appear to be relatively highly radioresistant. Doses of up to 50 Gy seem to have no significant effect on the ability of granulocytes to phagocytize and kill bacteria through the oxygen-dependent mechanism. Doses as high as 100 Gy also seem to have no effect on chemotactically directed motility.[49] More detailed studies on the oxygen-dependent killing mechanism, however, have introduced some doubts regarding the radioresistance of granulocytes with respect to oxygen-dependent bacterial killing mechanisms. Radiation dosages that vary from 25 to 50 Gy have been shown to cause variable decreases in superoxide anion generation, varying from 5% to as much as 70% in reduction capability.

The most effective method of prevention available for transfusion-related GVHD is clearly the irradiation of blood products to be administered to high-risk susceptible persons. Careful evaluation of clinical susceptibility, followed by the use of irradiated products, where otherwise the viable lymphocyte content would fall into a high-risk category, offers the best preventive technique. Some categories of patients clearly demand a universality of irradiated products, where cellular blood components are concerned. Thus, bone marrow transplant recipients receive only irradiated blood products, with the possible exception of fresh frozen plasma or cryoprecipitate, if these should be required for any reason. Similarly, patients with congenital immunodeficiency syndromes, and most particularly the severe combined immunodeficiency syndrome, should receive only irradiated cellular blood products. In other cases, the potential risk should be evaluated clinically, after which an appropriate product can be selected. With regard to the transfusion of newborns, there is no evidence that the use of frozen, deglycerolized RBCs in saline suspension with adjusted hematocrit carries any real risk of inducing GVHD. Conversely, products used for whole blood exchange transfusion should be carefully selected to avoid the possible presence of a critical mass of viable lymphocytes. Thus, the use of irradiated RBC products, whole blood, or reconstituted frozen, deglycerolized RBCs with fresh frozen plasma all appear to be safe for use in exchange transfusion, including that of premature newborns. Babies who have received intrauterine transfusions for HDN prior to delivery should be transfused exclusively with irradiated products.

A recent recommendation of the American Association of Blood Banks (1990) addresses the question of directed blood donors and the transfusion of "first-order" relatives. First-order relatives include parents, children, and siblings. The transfusion of blood products channeled from children into parents, from parents into children, or from siblings into each other should never be undertaken without prior irradiation of the products. This warning excludes fresh frozen plasma or cryoprecipitate. We have already learned that the establishment of transfusion-related GVHD is dependent on both HLA similarity and HLA disparity between recipient and donor. Since even the little difference of 1 HLA antigen (or even a non-HLA antigen or antigens) can enable a successfully grafted lymphocyte population to reject its host, the wisdom of this rule concerning near relatives is clearly obvious.

The necessary dosage of radiation required to be effected must still be settled. Generally, a dose of 15 Gy is regarded as adequate if mixed lymphocyte culture response is taken as the determinant criterion. Conversely, if mitogenic response is considered to be significant in this context, then higher dosages would clearly be necessary. A reasonable compromise of 25 Gy for all cellular blood products would seem to be acceptable. Further research into radiation dosage may be necessary before any definitive answers covering all cellular blood products can be obtained. In the meantime, large blood centers, particularly those dealing with bone marrow transplantation patients and those with various kinds of immunodeficiency (from congenital to acquired), should be able to provide irradiated products without delay whenever requested. Furthermore, these particular blood centers should offer the appropriate availability of either a Cesium$^{137}$ or Cobalt$^{60}$ gamma source.

## REFERENCES

1. Howland PV. Prevention of transfusion-associated graft-vs-host disease. Arch Pathol Lab Med. 1989;113:285.
2. Slavin RE, Santos GW. The graft-vs-host reaction in man after bone marrow transplantation: pathology, pathogenesis, clinical features and implications. Clin Immunol Immunopathol. 1973;1:472.
3. Simes MA, Koskimides S. Chronic graft-vs-host disease after blood transfusion confirmed by incompatible HLA antigens in bone marrow. Lancet. 1982;1:42.
4. Sakakibara T, Juiji T. Post-transfusion graft-vs-host disease and open heart surgery. Lancet. 1986;2:1099.
5. Ito K, Yoshida H, Yanaghashi K, et al. Change of HLA phenotype in post-operative erythrodermia. Lancet. 1988;1:413.
6. Shimoda T. On postoperative erythrodermia. Geka. 1955;17:487.
7. Aoki Y, Nakamura H, Sakabirara Y, et al. Probable graft-vs-host reaction following massive blood transfusion in an aged patient with postoperative aortic aneurysm: a case report. Nippon Naika Gakkai Zasshi. 1984;73:99.
8. Ino T, Matsura A, Takanashi R, et al. GVH-like syndrome following blood transfusion in patients undergoing cardiac operations. Geka. 1986;48:706.
9. Juiji T, Takahashi T. National survey on postoperative cases of GVH-like syndrome: the 1986 Report for Blood Research Project. Tokyo, Japan: Ministry of Health and Welfare; 1986.
10. Thomas ED, Storb R, Clift RA, et al. Bone marrow transplantation. N Engl J Med. 1975;292:832.
11. Graw RG, Buckner CD, Whang-Peng J, et al. Complication of bone-marrow transplantation: graft-vs-host disease resulting from chronic myelogenous leukemia leukocyte transfusion. Lancet. 1970;2:338.
12. Brubaker DB. Human post-transfusion graft-vs-host disease. Vox Sang. 1983;45:401.
13. Hathaway WE, Githens JH, Blackburn WR, et al. Aplastic anemia, histiocystosis and erythrodermia in immunologically deficient children. N Engl J Med. 1965;273:953.
14. Hathaway WE, Fulginiti DA, Pierce CW, et al. Graft-vs-host reaction following a single blood transfusion. JAMA. 1967;201:139.
15. Niethammer D, Goldmann SF, Glad HD, et al. Graft-vs-host reaction after blood transfusion in a patient with cellular immunodeficiency: the role of histocompatibility testing. J Pediatr. 1979;132:43.

16. Leitma SF, Holland PV. Irradiation of blood products: indications and guidelines. Transfusion. 1985;25:293.
17. Mayer KT. Transfusion support of leukemia and oncology patients. Clin Haematol. 1984;14:93.
18. Park BH, Good RA, Gate J, et al. Fatal graft-vs-host reaction following transfusion of allogeneic blood and plasma in infants with combined immunodeficiency disease. Transplant Proc. 1974;6:385.
19. Douglas SD, Fudenberg HH. Graft-vs-host reaction in Wiskott-Aldrich syndrome: antimortem diagnosis of human GVH in an immunologic deficient disease. Vox Sang. 1969;16:172.
20. Rubenstein A, Rad J, Cotter H, et al. Unusual combined immunodeficiency syndrome exhibiting kappa-IgD paraproteinemia, residual gut-immunity and graft-vs-host reaction after plasma infusion. Acta Paediatr Scand. 1973;62:365.
21. Seemayer TA, Bolane PR. Thymic involution mimicking thymic dysplasia: a consequence of transfusion-induced graft-vs-host disease in a premature infant. Arch Pathol Lab Med. 1980;104:141.
22. Naiman JL, Punnett HH, Lischener HW, et al. Possible graft-vs-host reaction after intrauterine transfusion for Rh erythroblastosis fetalis. N Engl J Med. 1969;281:697.
23. Parkman R, Mosier D, Umanski I, et al. Graft-vs-host disease in two newborns after repeated exchange transfusions for hemolytic disease of the newborn. N Engl J Med. 1974;290:359.
24. Bohm N, Kleime W, Enzel U. Graft-vs-host disease in two newborns after repeated blood transfusions because of rhesus incompatibility. Bertr Pathol. 1977;160:381.
25. Hathaway WE, Brangler RW, Nelson TL, et al. Aplastic anemia and alymphocytosis in an infant with hypogammaglobulinemia, graft-vs-host reaction? J Pediatr. 1966;68:713.
26. Von Flidener V, Higby VJ, Kim U. Graft-vs-host reaction following blood transfusion. Am J Med. 1982;72:951.
27. Mathe G, Bernard J, De Vries MJ, et al. Nouveaux essais de greffe de moelle osseuse homologue apres irradiation totale chez des enfants atteints de leucemie aige en remission: le probleme due syndrome secondaire chez l'homme. Rev Hematol. 1960;15:115.
28. Murphy ML, Helson L. Chemotherapy of metastatic neuroblastoma stage IV. ASCO Abs Tr. 1977;285:338.
29. Woods WG, Luben DM. Fatal graft-vs-host disease following a blood transfusion in a child with neuroblastoma. Pediatrics. 1981;67:217.
30. Kennedy JS, Rickets RR. Fatal graft-vs-host disease in a child with neuroblastoma following a blood transfusion. J Pediatr Surg. 1986;21:1108.
31. Labotka RJ, Radvany R. Graft-vs-host disease in rhabdomyosarcoma following transfusion with non-irradiated blood products. Med Pediatr Oncol. 1985;13:101.
32. Schmidmeier W, Feill W, Gebhart W, et al. Fatal graft-vs-host reaction following granulocyte transfusion. Blut. 1982;45:115.
33. Fauci AS, Macher M, Longo DL, et al. Acquired immunodeficiency syndrome: epidemiologic, clinical, immunologic and therapeutic considerations. Ann Intern Med. 1984;100:92.
34. Lowenthal RW, Goldman JM, Buskard NA. Granulocyte transfusions in treatment of infections in patients with acute leukemia and aplastic anemia. Lancet. 1975;1:35.
35. Burns LJ, Westberg MW, Burns CP, et al. Acute graft-vs-host disease resulting from normal donor blood transfusions. Acta Haematol. 1984;71:270.
36. Van Belken V. Transfusion and transplantation. Isr J Med Sci. 1965;1:879.
37. Bornes DWH, Toutt JD. Splenic protection: the cellular hypothesis. In: Baca B, ed. Radiology Symposium. Woburn, Mass: Butterworths; 1954:134.
38. Syskind GW, Thomas L. Studies on the runting syndrome in newborn mice. J Exp Med. 1958;110:511.

39. De Witte C. Personal communication, 1990.
40. Mathe G, Bernard J, Schwarzenberg R, et al. Essai de traitement de sujets atteints de leucemie aigue en remission par irradiation totale suive de transfusion de moelle osseuse homologue. Rev Fr Etudes Clin Biol. 1959;4:675.
41. Graze PR, Goale PR. Chronic graft-vs-host disease: a syndrome of disordered immunity. Am J Med. 1979;66:611.
42. Fagiolo E, D'Addosio AM. First-transfusion graft-vs-host disease (GVHD) immunopathology and prevention. Haematologica. 1985;70:62.
43. Weiden P. Graft-vs-host disease following blood transfusions. Arch Intern Med. 1984;14:115.
44. Sprent J, Anderson RE, Miller JF. Radiosensitivity of T and B lymphocytes, II: effect of irradiation on response of T-cells to alloantigens. Eur J Immunol. 1974;4:204.
45. Crowley JT, Skrabut EM, Valeri CR. Immunocompetent lymphocytes in previously frozen washed red cells. Vox Sang. 1974;26:513.
46. Valerius NH, Johansen KS, Nielsen OS, et al. Effect of in vitro X-irradiation on lymphocyte and granulocyte function. Scand J Haematol. 1981;27:9.
47. Moroff G, George VM, Siegl AM, et al. The influence of irradiation on stored platelets. Transfusion. 1986;26:453.
48. Button LM, Wolff WC, Newburger PE, et al. The effects of irradiation on blood components. Transfusion. 1981;21:419.
49. Ramirez AM, Woodfield DG, Scott R, et al. High potassium levels in stored irradiated blood. Transfusion. 1987;27:444.
50. Holley TR, Van Epps DE, Harvey RL. Effects of high doses of radiation on human neutrophil chemotaxis, phagocytosis and morphology. Am J Pathol. 1974;75:61.

# INDEX

*Numbers in **boldface** refer to pages on which figures appear; numbers followed by a t indicate tabular material.*

## D

## H

## O



## P

## S



## T

## U



## V



## W



## Y